Pippa Publications

Los Angeles – Buenos Aires   2012

Dr. David S. Cantor is a gastroenterologist in Los Angeles, California.

He had been Assistant Professor of Medicine at UC Davis, Clinical Professor of Medicine at University of Southern California, President of the Medical Staff at Huntington Hospital, Pasadena, CA, President of the Southern Society for Gastrointestinal Endoscopy and President of the Pasadena Medical Society.

He worked in private practice and clinical research. He has published a Textbook of Gastroenterology and Hepatology and 50 scientific papers.

He has been a co-founder and Editor of Acta Gastroenterologica LatinoAmericana.

He co-founded Health Alert a Medical Newsletter.

Dr. Cantor has been awarded with the James N. Gamble award in 2007 among other distinctions

THE BOOK OF GOOD HEALTH

DESTROYING MYTHS, LIES AND DECEPTIONS. REAFFIRMING TRUTHS TO ACHIEVE TOTAL WELLNESS

DAVID S. CANTOR M.D.

This book is available in Amazon.com under 'The Book of Good Health by David Cantor', Kindle and selected Bookstores

To my family, the source of my commitment

To my patients, the source of my inspiration

Foreword

When I was looking for a publisher for this book, the first question asked was in what way it was different from the thousands of other health books that are available in the marketplace.

Most of the other books are aimed at helping people attain wellbeing, but none are comprehensive enough to provide all the answers because good health is multifaceted. The only way to achieve wellness, to prevent disease and to delay the onset of infirmities is to eat well (Nutrition), to be physically fit (Training), to be happy (Stress Management), to take the least amount of medication (Drugs and other paraphernalia), to avoid getting sick (Prevention) and to live a 'pastoral life' in a non-pastoral world. In this sense *The Book of Good Health* is several books in one.

Our internal wiring is changing; we used to eat to survive and now we eat to indulge. The air we breathe poisons our body, anxiety maims us, and medications are therapeutic but also toxic.

The book supplies the information needed to apply the extraordinary advances of medicine judiciously. In this way one may challenge the ills of civilization and return to a better, simple more rewarding life.

Table of Contents:

Introduction

INTRODUCTION

On July 2, 2009 Jon Stewart, the host of Comedy Central's *The Daily Show* was interviewing documentary filmmaker Robert Kenner about his movie *Food, Inc.*, which denounced the practices of the food industry and the role of the US Department of Agriculture and the Food and Drug Administration in allowing these questionable practices. Mr. Kenner made some revelations about the harmful consequences of the food we consume and the lack of effective controls regarding safety. Mr. Stewart, playing devil's advocate and with his trademark bluntness, asked him to explain why we are not dying earlier, since life expectancy in the United States is better today than it ever has been. He was right; according to the U.S. Census Bureau the projection for the year 2010 is that we will live 78.3 years as an average (75.7 for males and 80.8 for females). Still, life expectancy is a very poor health indicator, impacted excessively by technology-driven life prolonging mechanisms that do not take into account quality of life. Length of life would be a great indicator if combined with quality of life. Today we have the technical capability to keep people alive longer than ever before. We use respirators to make patients breathe, gastric tubes to feed them, and all kind of devices to prolong life, and we do this very well. For practical purposes it would be better to measure quality-adjusted life expectancy.

In Bhutan, a country with a rich and unique cultural heritage nestled in the Eastern Himalayas, instead of using the Gross National Product as an indicator of the condition of the country, they use the Gross National Happiness Index (GNHI). This concept was first created by their former King Signa Singye Wangchuck and although at the beginning it was not taken seriously, today it is an acceptable indicator, being proposed by Tony Blair in England and Nicholas Sarkozy in

France as a guide to assess the wellness of the population. The metrics being used as part of the GNHI are economic, physical, mental and environmental as well as political, social and workplace factors. Canada and other European countries are also seriously considering the adoption of the GNHI as a quantitative and qualitative benchmark to assess the welfare of their people. Bhutan ranks among the eight happiest countries in the world, while the United States is 113, a fact that suggests that there is no correlation between per capita income and advances in technology and life enjoyment.

Wellbeing and happiness depend on many factors, such as socio-economic status, housing, literacy, environment, family, genetics, and health—all of which are among the prongs of a more ample fork. Health is the most important because without it the others become irrelevant.

The United States is a well-endowed country, the richest country in human history. It is an economic power and its inhabitants have one of the best standards of living in the world. It is a fierce protector of freedom of speech, free enterprise, and civil liberties, achievements that are always in peril and in need of preservation and renewal. This may be seen as a blessing but it is also a curse when myths, lies and deceptions in the health field are left unchecked and uncontested, creating an unwholesome population with insalubrious habits. Common sense and verifiable facts have yielded to the might of individuals and corporations who, in the single-minded quest of making money, are changing our habits and our way of life. They encourage consumption and manipulate our thoughts; they influence our lifestyle and create illusions to maintain their full coffers. The end result is that we get distracted by false promises about the quality of what we eat; we get lost in phony shortcuts to achieve wellness and end up not being who we should be or who we want to be. The power and efficiency of advertising becomes dicey when the same communication tools used to convey the virtues of a car or a pair of jeans are used to peddle medications, non-substantive diets, unneeded surgeries, insalubrious foods and untested medical treatments, to name a few of the culprits in perpetuating unhealthy habits. When marketing influences what we wear or what we drive, the consequences may not be detrimental but when it comes to health issues those machinations jeopardize our wellbeing, or kill us.

Our wealth as a country has started to show in our sizes. We are a nation of fat people. According to the Center for Disease and Control Prevention (CDC), 34 percent of adults aged 20 and over and 32 percent of children are overweight. In more dramatic terms 144 million Americans are obese, the dire consequences of which are the development of Type 2 diabetes, cardiovascular disease, hypertension, stroke, cancer of all types, mental illness, degenerative disease, back pain, neurological ailments, genetic defects and other infirmities prevalent in the United States.

A multitude of causes contribute to this bizarre disparagement of our most treasured value: our health. The responsibility for maiming our wellbeing is shared by individuals and corporations who have an economic interest in perpetuating this stance. Fortunately others, persons and institutions, have a strong interest in setting the record straight and work very hard to enlighten people and leading the way to change our lifestyle so we can achieve optimal health.

Can we decrease the frequency of the ills and harm produced by the reckless and negligent actions of the food industry and the pharmaceutical companies? Yes, we can. Can we manage and control their deeds and avoid premature infirmity and death? Yes, we can.

In this book we add our voice to the challenges of our time affecting our wellbeing by providing data, information and facts about the distortion of health issues. We tear down the fairytales, analyze the legends, point to falsehoods and denounce the fabrications that surround the health paradigm. Dishonesty and mendacity have no place in this arena. It is not an easy task because the forces to overcome are everywhere, disguised with different clothes. It is not only greed from others trampling us; it is also our critical internal needs for safety and comfort that allow magical thinking and delusions to prevail.

And yet, we are not doomed, because despite the enormity of the task, the power to change is within us. Already our efforts have made smoking less common. There are 46 million smokers in the United States. Smoking causes 440,000 preventable, premature deaths every year. Thanks to efforts by the government, citizens and scientific groups like the American Heart Association, the consumption of tobacco has decreased by half in the last three decades (tobacco companies still take advantage of more flexible world legislation in developing countries, where cigarette consumption is increasing at a rate of 3.4% yearly). These statistics show several things: campaigns to stop the use of tobacco are extremely effective and when localities, state or the federal government regulate its use (for instance by not allowing casual smoking to be shown in movies or banning the sale of cigarettes near schools), they accomplish what they intend to do; inversely, in developing countries, where regulations are lax and corruption prevalent, consumption keeps increasing. Believe it or not, 15 billion cigarettes are smoked daily in the world, a staggering number, taking into consideration that the world population is less than 8 billion people. The British, American and Japanese tobacco corporations dominate almost the entire tobacco market.

The formidable task of preventing disease by eliminating external factors, such as smoking, can also be achieved in other areas like eliminating harmful food, avoiding unnecessary intake of prescription and non-prescription medications and minimizing exposure to toxins and other injurious agents.

The foundation for achieving good health is simple and it is disconcerting that we deviate from the road of wellbeing so often and so willingly. This book is a step-by-step guide to understanding the why, where and when of what we do wrong so we can choose to do the right thing. There are no magic solutions, standard recipes or fairytale formulas to feel good and stay strong and healthy. It is rather a matter of changing habits, discarding biases, stopping the pernicious influence of the merchants of deception, and learning to separate the grains of truth from the lies.

We have the power to transform what appears set and inflexible. We have a voice in making sure that medication errors are brought down from one million occurrences a year to smaller numbers, that opportunistic infections will not kill us when we are in a hospital and that hospital falls injuring thousands of patients can be prevented. We have a voice in demanding health reform to include everybody and provide proper education to stay well.

So simple and yet so challenging. If you think when you are eating a nice piece of chicken you are nourishing yourself, think again: you may be consuming a lot of nasty chemicals. If you think that the thousands of dollars you are spending to make your back pain disappear are well spent, think again; you are probably wasting your money. If you believe that the Food and Drug Administration has already taken all the safeguards needed to make sure that the medications you take are harmless and effective, you are plain wrong.

Knowledge will empower you to avoid being at the mercy of the racketeers, the ones who are poisoning your food and pushing you to take needless medications. If you are afflicted with an ailment we will teach how to treat it judiciously and what measures you can take to improve your health and improve the quality of your life.

We can encapsulate the prescription for good health in few words: maintain a good state of nutrition by eating a well-balanced diet, low in cholesterol and saturated fat; get sufficient sleep; have periodic medical and dental examinations; stop bad habits, exercise regularly and don't take medications when they are not needed. This is your individual responsibility; nobody can do this for you. Society in turn needs to make sure that people are guaranteed a home, education, medical care and recreation and good transportation, similar to the second Bill of Rights proposed by President Roosevelt but never enacted.

And yet so difficult... You are probably one of the millions of people eating too much fat, the wrong kind of carbohydrates and too little proteins, not getting enough rest, seeking medical help in the wrong places and not exercising in a meaningful way.

I wrote this book to have a chat with the public as a way of prolonging my lifelong dialogue with my patients. I put pen to paper in a time of a profound economic crisis comparable to the Great Depression, and this gave me a sense of urgency to tell the readers that they should not wrongly use the system of medicine as in times past and thereby making the remedy the disease. There are 45 million people without health insurance and another 25 million underinsured. They, like the rest of us, need to avoid the wrong tools in the quest to stay healthy. Huge budgets are being squandered and abused by bureaucracies and fraud, preventing a rational use of our common wealth.

This is what you should not expect from this book: another diet guidebook, like the ones that you read and abandon (only 2% of people are able to lose weight and keep it off); wonder drugs and miracle cures; promises to make you look 60 years old when you are 80; rather, we will help you to stay a healthy, energetic and happy 80.

It is time to understand that contrary to popular perception, aging is not an inexorable loss of mental and physical capacity. It is true that some functions may deteriorate, like memory, capacity to remember names and solve mathematical problems and others, but our brains may compensate by making us connect better with our emotions. After all, the elders are still the wiser members of their tribes. Look around: Clint Eastwood is 79 and still directing wonderful movies;

Bruce Springsteen, now 60 years old, is delighting us with his music; Winston Churchill, the notable politician won the Nobel Prize in Literature at the age of 79; Mother Teresa worked incessantly until her death at age 87; Rita Levi-Montalcini, who won the Nobel Prize in medicine, is still very active and was 103 years old on April 22, 2012; and on and on. It is not that they are special people with special aptitudes but rather that they discarded the bias that aging is a process of mental and physical deterioration. Dr. Florin Dolcos, a member of the Alberta Cognitive Neuroscience Group, showed that old people can actually manage how much attention they give to negative situations so they are less upset by them. He reached this conclusion by exploring how the brains of old people work in issues like perception, attention, learning, memory, language, decision making, emotion and development. He demonstrated that the amygdala, a brain region involved in emotion detection, and the anterior cingulate cortex, a brain region involved in emotion control, have an increased interaction that gets better with aging. This implies that aging is not a total degenerative process but rather one where there are areas of definite improvement.

We need to engage seriously in your pursuit of good health. It is not only a physical but also a spiritual mission.

This is the promise: do the right thing and your cells will look much younger than those of people who are much younger than you but are engaged in insalubrious habits. A group of scientists from the Saarland University of Hamburg found that the telomeres of the white cells of active young adults look similar in length to those of middle-aged athletes and better than sedentary subjects.

Some basic concepts about telomeres: Tissues are composed of cells; cells contain organelles, one of which is called the nucleus. The nucleus contains chromosomes, which contain all the genetic information that is passed from parents to children.

Cells divide and form new cells to assure growth and development. When they duplicate they make sure that each daughter cell get half of the genetic material so they will pass the information from one generation to the next. Each chromosome has a protective cap called telomere. This telomere loses a little bit of length each time a cell divides, and when it becomes too short the chromosome reaches a critical length and can no longer replicate, meaning that a cell has aged, which is the same as saying the body has aged. But if the enzyme telomerase, which is essential to the preservation of the telomere, is again activated, the cell will continue to grow and divide. In other words, to a certain point the aging process will stop or be delayed.

Telomeres are in a way a marker of cell age. Researchers found that sedentary people have telomeres that are on average 40 percent shorter than the ones from active young adults, while middle-aged runners had telomeres than were only 10 percent shorter than young runners. Another study by Thomas LaRocca from the University of Colorado showed that subjects between the ages of 55 and 72 who had a maximum aerobic capacity (a marker of physical fitness) have longer telomeres. In other words, regular exercise improves the quality of our cells.

I always have been surprised that in certain important areas of work one does not need a formal education—for example, politics. A person may become a senator or president of a nation without having been schooled in international affairs, economy, sociology, logic and other disciplines—and yet we entrust our destiny to them. One cannot imagine a high rise building being developed without certified engineers and architects. And yet in an area as important as health, education is missing on the development, maintenance and preservation of our wellbeing. It is time to provide everybody with knowledge, so they can develop the skills to be the best they can, physically and spiritually. It is time to become the engineers of our own health.

Before I close this chapter let me share with you some of my thoughts. I have been a physician for more than 50 years, working at the beginning of my career in research and then as a clinical gastroenterologist. I have helped the poor, the rich, the destitute and the opulent. My patients have visited me more than 250,000 times and in this undertaking I gave as much as I could. In the process I learned a great deal about human beings by sharing their angst, fears, hopes and their happiness. I have influenced them by being a good listener and by my everlasting optimism. Medicine is my faith and my commitment, so I wrote this book to help others in being well and staying healthy. Good advice is out there and today, in the era of the Internet, more reachable than ever. But bad guidance is also there and at close range. So I felt that I may make a difference by helping the public understand where their ills are coming from and how to fight them in a sensible and judicious way.

Anecdotes in this book have been told to make a point but never to enthrone them as a truth. All the assertions in this book have a foundation in rigorous science, research studies and proven epidemiological data. I have quoted word by word certain studies
that are in the public domain when I considered that they conveyed the message clearly and better than I could. My task has been greatly facilitated by the Internet, which gave me the opportunity to sieve among thousands of scientific studies. As a physician I have full access to scientific papers. I decided to quote those that are more relevant to the reader.

My patients have been always my best teachers, and no pleasure has been greater in my life than serve and honor them. This book is another way of answering their questions and continuing my service.

Chapter 1:

NUTRITION – PART 1

A TALE OF TWO CITIES

It was the best of times; it was the worst of times…

1

It is not a delusion. It actually was that way when I was a child. As we heard the man shouting 'milk, milk, fresh milk' and the sound of a clapper striking a bell, my mother would give me a large empty cooking pot and send me out to fetch a full load. The man and the cow would pace slowly on the cobblestone street. He would unpack a small three-legged stool from his back and milk the cow, squirting the cow's udder with his bare hands, fill the pot, decide that it rendered about a gallon and charge me 10 cents. We lived in a quaint middle class neighborhood and were lucky to have the provider of milk wandering around the streets with his trusty cow. Other food suppliers were also at hand.

The fruit and vegetable vendor walked side by side with the pony pulling a cart full with fresh produce. He would stop at each corner, waiting for the neighbors to gather and buy his cargo.

The *Panaderia* was the sanctuary of bread, cakes, pastries, candies and chocolates, all of them cooked on-site. The smell of fresh bread permeated to the streets. Bread was cooked three times a day for freshness, and we used to go there twice a day to get it just off the oven.

The butcher would slice the meats quickly, but not before inquiring how we were going to cook it (grilled, baked or boiled?) and how many people would be eating, after which time he would chose the cut and the quantity.

The rest of the food we bought in the *Almacen,* the general store. Edibles came in big containers and were seldom pre-packed. If we wanted a kilogram of sugar it was procured from a large sackcloth, scooped out and wrapped in an old newspaper sheet. Flour and rice were also divided at time of purchase.

We ate four meals a day. For breakfast, we had *café con leche* (one quarter coffee and three quarters hot milk in a large cup with three to four teaspoonfuls of sugar), fresh bread with a tantalizing aroma and texture, with a generous spread of butter and jam. At 'tea time' we added pastries. Lunch and dinner almost always included beef, which was abundant and cheap in Argentina; the variation was in the cuts and the preparation. Steaks were grilled or fried. Beef was either stewed or cooked in the oven. Fish, chicken, pork or turkey was eaten more sparingly because these meats were expensive. As side dishes, we had eggs, mashed potatoes with plenty of butter or maize oil, rice and vegetables. To drink, we had tap water or carbonated water in soda siphons, delivered at home twice a week, and inexpensive table wine. Pasta was usually homemade and sauces were prepared from fresh tomatoes. For dessert there was fresh fruit. Daily cooking was simple. Mother would cook sophisticated ethnic dishes, mostly on holidays, when the family would gather around the big table.

Nutrition, cholesterol, low fat diet, excess salt, calories, protein, carbohydrates or fat were never topics of conversation. Milk and bread were implicitly held in the highest regard, indispensable, always present, a gift from God; the rest of what we ate was a cornucopia, provided by the generous fertile pampas. Foodstuffs needed to be consumed promptly to avoid spoilage; there were no electric refrigerators. Perishables were kept in a wooden icebox lined with tin, which at its base had a drip pan to catch the water from the melting ice bar. Provisions were renewed every two to three days.

We consumed all organic food, but too much fat, mainly from meats and butter. Paradoxically, obesity was infrequent.

The place was Buenos Aires, the time early 1940s.

2

My grandchildren were coming to visit from Miami. We needed to replenish our food supplies. These kids don't eat, they gorge. My wife gave me a list of groceries and off I went. I drove my car to the supermarket. Parking was easy. I entered the place: the landscape was impressive. The store was on one very large level, well lighted with clean, shiny floors. The display of produce, meats, dairy, beverages and household products was striking. Pyramids of fruits were still perspiring from the recent mist provided by a hose. But wait a minute—where is the smell of fresh fruit? Now I am in the bakery section. Where is the smell of fresh bread? I feel like paraphrasing the Argentinean poet Baldomero Fernandez Moreno, who wrote, "Seventy balconies there are in this building/ seventy balconies and not one flower/ to its inhabitants, Lord what happens? They hate the smell, hate the color." Something like, "Supermarket full of things/ to its inhabitants, Lord, what happens? They hate the smell, hate the flavor."

My first visit to an American supermarket was in Mount Rainier, Maryland, in 1959. Coming from Argentina, where they were nonexistent, I was struck by the ingenuity of the place. It was the first time that I saw a shopping cart, my first

20

practice with self-service and the novelty of noticing all kinds of food and household products under one roof. Shopping hours were from six in the morning till midnight, impossible in many countries where strict labor laws restricted working hours. There were no counters, just shelves. For the first time we became active participants in the buying process, since assistants were available only by demand. For us, the supermarket experience was a topic of conversation as important as the visit to the Smithsonian, the Lincoln Memorial and other highlights of the city.

I am still amazed at the transformation of these markets; today we can find cheeses from all over the world, fish from Vietnam, wines from Chile, olives from Greece and the best of the best from the rest of the world. Before the Internet, it was the supermarket that interconnected the planet.

Today one can avoid a long line at the cashier stand by using a self-service checkout machine, where one weighs the produce, scans the merchandise and pays with cash or credit card, which represents the epitome of self-service and a demonstration of the confidence of the supermarkets toward their clients.

Going back to our story:

I started in the dairy section to buy the first item on the list, milk. There were many variations: non-fat, 1 percent, 2 percent, whole, flavored, organic with or without added vitamin A and D, predigested for those with lactase deficiency and goat, soy, almond, rice and hemp milks. Second on the list was orange juice. The alternatives were many: just squeezed, from concentrate, mixed with strawberry juice and/or others. Cereals: I counted more than ninety-two variations. There were so many options that I gave up and called my wife on my cell for guidance. Forty-five minutes later I was back home with six bags of groceries. She smelled the tomatoes and complained, "These are tasteless; I told you to buy the ones on the vine." When she got to the cereals, another protest: "These have too much sugar." Then four more grievances: "The fruits are not ripe"; "Tilapia was farm grown and I asked you to buy fresh fish"; "meat was not lean"; "butter was supposed to be unsalted." Abundance makes life complicated.

The place was Los Angeles, the time early 2010.

3

In 2012 Buenos Aires resembles Los Ángeles. National and foreign corporations have built huge supermarkets practically undistinguishable from their American counterparts, but in Argentina you still can find thousands of small retail suppliers of food. The bakery, the grocery store, and the farmers' markets remain well established, treasured and respected. Owners and clients call each other by their first names and greet each other with a kiss on the cheek. Buenos Aires has a European flavor. People cherish eating; the art of cooking is a frequent topic of conversation; restaurants are mindful about the food they serve and careful about the ambiance. Even in times of economic crisis, eateries are packed. Industrialization of food is looked down upon and yet because of their ease and comfort, supermarkets are visited frequently. Sophisticated consumers know that not all olive oil is the same; that meat is different if the cattle have been allowed to pasture in the fields instead of being fed with corn in cages; wine is a matter of grapes and processing and not marketing. This applies to all victuals. When it comes to food, people have a certain degree of sophistication. Argentineans are proud that the grapes for Malbec wine grow only in their soil, that the flavor of the meat is exceptional because cows are fed with the grass that is unique to their prairies. The restaurant chefs are mostly descendants of Italians and Spaniards who have improved the legacy of their ancestors and are part of the cultural scenery of the city.

Food is an object of idolization, with a strong cultural meaning that puts the brakes on the invasion of processed foods, artificial nutrients, genetically engineered fruits, hybrid vegetables, etc. Tourists go to Argentina to eat beef, which is plentiful, tasty and relatively cheap, and to drink wines from Mendoza or Salta, which are considered among the best in the world; friends meet for hours around the dining table either at home or eateries. There is always a restaurant around the corner, from the homey to the sophisticated.

Was 1940 the golden age of food in Argentina and the model that that we should follow today? Should we go back to the way of cooking that the rainbow of European immigrants brought to their new land? During the first 40 years of the last century people predominantly came from Spain, Italy and eastern European countries, seeking solace in the promising lands of South America; they came with few personal belongings but with strong cultural baggage. The settlers became rapidly assimilated to their new home while the natives adopted many of their good traditions. When it came to food, Argentineans learned from the Italians how to cook pasta and pizza, seafood from the Spaniards, stew from the Hungarians. Today the Argentinean cuisine is a garland of the best dishes from most of the world.

Food was nutritional and tasty, without chemicals or preservatives. Pasteurization was introduced at the end of the nineteenth century but was not universally adopted until the mid 1940s. Fruit and vegetables compelled their consumption while fresh to avoid decay. Cows roamed freely in the farm and ate the grass that grew easily in the pampas. Irrigation systems were not needed because of frequent rains. Food was plentiful, relatively inexpensive and very appetizing. Consequently, in spite of Buenos Aires being a modern metropolitan city, meals were similar to the ones of people living in rural areas. Today things are different. In most rural areas, which comprise more than 50 percent of the country, people consume what is produced locally by small farmers, or from nearby provinces and seldom from neighboring countries. This food is truly organic. In contrast, in big cities some of the foodstuff comes from abroad and manufacturing, processing, marketing and distribution is similar to the food of industrialized countries.

Tuscany in Italy is an extensive area of valleys, plains and mountains, with few large cities and lots of small villages surrounded by fields blossoming with agricultural products. Like in Buenos Aires in the 40s there are grocers everywhere, but like modern cities, tens of thousands of products are also gathered in modern markets.

Italians and Argentineans have the convenience of the supermarket and at the same time access to organic edibles. In contrast, in the US processed foods are more prominent and ninety-five percent of meat comes from industrial plants. People in big metropolitan areas seek organic produce in specialty stores or in the occasional farmers' market.

When food consumption in a country starts resembling the American model, people start getting similar infirmities. Ulcerative colitis and Crohn's disease, two chronic and at times severe conditions, were rare in Argentina in the fifties; now the incidences equal those in the United States.

Obesity in Argentina (or Latin America) was not a problem in the past, while now it is slowly emerging as a dreaded condition, although not to the extent that prevails in the United States.

In France, in spite of smoking being so prevalent and diet being rich in saturated fat, people have a low incidence of coronary artery disease. There is no definitive explanation for this phenomenon; the theory is that they consume less junk food, drink more red wine, have a more active lifestyle, or a combination of all.

This brings me to the core of this chapter: Are we, as claimed by investigative reporter Eric Schlosser in his book *Fast Food Nation: The Dark Side of the All-American Meal* and other writings, eating the wrong stuff due mainly to the current industrial food system?

Michael Pollan, another author concerned with our eating habits, wrote a best seller *The Omnivore's Dilemma,* a controversial book. He investigated the procedures in the food production system, from agricultural practices to the final food products, providing evidence that the content, due to manipulation and additives, is deleterious to our health.

In *The End of Overeating: Taking Control of the Insatiable American Appetite* Dr. David Kessler, a pediatrician, lawyer, author and past commissioner of the Food and Drug Administration explains why we tend to eat the wrong stuff and how we can break the cycle of eating too much of the wrong thing.

These three books give support to the assumption that people are eating the wrong stuff simply because they don't know what they are eating. Furthermore, as will be later explained, eating processed food sets the body into a frenzy to eat more of it, entering into a catch-22 situation. As a result people get sick and many die.

Over the last 40 years our eating habits have gone through a cultural and sociological transformation, forcing us to consume food not guided by our instincts and desires but by the design of external forces that are conspiring to make us eat what they produce to increase the profitability of their corporations. By doing so, they are changing the anatomy and the physiology of the human body and causing the appearance of infirmities that we never experienced before. This may sound outlandish and barely credible to the reader but in the next chapters I will illustrate how we are sharing the fate of animals subjected to certain experiments in the laboratory and why by doing so we are inviting a myriad of illness to maim us, illnesses which were infrequent 50 years ago, above all obesity, a calamity which triggers all kinds of ailments.

5

Obesity today is a national epidemic, an alarming condition associated with cardiovascular disease, hypertension, stroke, diabetes, arthritis and certain types of cancers like breast and gallbladder. It has become a public health problem on several fronts: it accelerates the appearance of disease (with all its dreadful implications at personal and family levels) and is a financial burden to society, since we all share the cost of medical care; the larger the number of sick people, the greater the premiums for medical insurance for the rest of us.

One way to reverse this trend is to understand obesity in a larger context and how we got to be a fat nation, learn its morbid connotations and ascertain the amazing mechanism that keeps a person in the normal range of weight and the consequences of its disruption.

High body fat is better understood by measuring the body mass index (BMI), which is the ratio of weight to height in metric measurements calculated by dividing one's weight by the square of one's height. It is more important to know our BMI than our weight and as important as other health parameters like blood pressure and cholesterol.

The National Institute of Health, the foremost government agency as it relates to biochemical and medical research, has established four BMI parameters: less than 18.5, **underweight**; 18.5 to 24.9, **healthy**; 25.0 to 29.9, **overweight** and more than 30, **obese**. To this we may add another category, **morbid obesity,** when the BMI is more than 40.

Patients who are overweight use more medical resources, impinging on the overall expense of medical care. This is critical because cost is a crucial component for access to medical care. The bottom line is that if we could control obesity we could substantially decrease the cost of health care. Obese people require special equipment like wider seats in airplanes, special tables to lie down for an X-ray or a CAT scan, and widening of revolving doors among other things, which create an additional cost to society.

It is an accepted truth that obesity is dreadful and a condition that needs to be addressed more seriously and yet despite all the scientific evidence, obesity is the center of a bizarre social controversy. Some fat people don't want to be patronized and resent the fact that society looks at them as social outcasts. To counter what they perceive as an attack they have organized in groups, have created slogans like' fat is beautiful', use the Internet to defend their stance, have found support in some doctors who don't see obesity as a health issue and quote articles published in medical journals that illustrate some beneficial aspects of obesity, like the ones that have shown that overweight patients on hemodyalisis do better than lean people or that they respond better than their counterparts to treatment of peripheral artery disease.

They claim that obesity is a trait and not a medical condition and feel attacked and perceive most of society having a spiteful attitude toward them, feel scorned and abused and resent jokes about obesity. Rubens, the sixteenth century artist, celebrated chubby females on canvas; at that time being somewhat overweight meant wealth and social status, as pallor did (only peasants and the working class were exposed to the sun and got a tan and were skinny because they did not have the resources to indulge in big meals). Rubens is their hero.

Although I sympathize with their cry to be accepted as 'normal' people, the defenders and champions of obesity who engage in an obesity acceptance crusade are producing more harm than good; it is one thing for fat people to genuinely campaign against being discriminated but it is a different story to push their agenda with all its alarming health implications. The facts are not in their favor. Research studies and epidemiological data have unequivocally shown that obesity is a health hazard.

Curiously, it was not until early in 1990 that it was brought to our attention that the weight of Americans has shown a dangerous upward trend. Katherine M. Flegal from the Centers for Disease Control (CDC) presented epidemiological data showing this trend. The medical community was for the first time made aware that the incidence of obesity was such that it was posing a serious health hazard. As always happens in America, when something becomes trendy, all kinds of crazes develop: business people took notice and established diet centers all around the country, the food industry developed palatable low calorie concoctions at a reasonable price. Diet gurus emerged like mushrooms; books were written and became best sellers overnight. The Scarsdale Medical Diet became a sensation for a few years (later when its author, Dr. Tarnower, was assassinated by his lover it regained fame). Dr. Atkins' Diet Revolution became popular in 1972 and franchises emerged to sell products associated with the program. Some people take advantage of certain situations using their ingenuity and entrepreneurship, some by honest means and others by deceitful deeds.

6

Numbers are eloquent: sixty-four percent of adults fall from the accepted criteria of normalcy (30 percent are overweight and 34 percent are obese, an important distinction) and more than 30 percent of children have a weight problem (in Louisiana 44 percent of kids are fat). People gain weight because of little physical activity and/or overeating. This used to be a predominant (not exclusive) American problem, but developed and undeveloped countries are catching up fast. Francis Delpeuch and others in their book *Globesity: A planet out of control* have shown that all continents are affected with the obesity malaise. This at first glance is surprising since one would expect that countries where the income per capita is very low would not have the resources to buy and eat food beyond their needs. But it is precisely the consumption of junk food, which is relatively inexpensive, that is the cause of excessive weight.

About 10 years ago I saw a 32 year old patient who was five–feet-eight and weighed 260 pounds. Among other ailments he had severe osteoporosis, a rather unusual condition in a young male patient. This condition is characterized by brittle bones due to reduced bone mineral density and it is not uncommon in women after menopause. I asked him to keep a diary of his food consumption for two weeks. His diet consisted mainly of carbohydrates, was hypercaloric, and was low in vitamins and calcium, which explained his condition. His weight was a hefty 260 and yet he was malnourished! This is a typical example of the fallacy of looking apparently healthy (like obese people) versus being healthy. The point is that many of us may appear in good physical condition, feel fit and yet may be harboring some medical condition, which underscores the need to have regular checkups, mainly if we are overweight. It is shocking that we take our car for service regularly and maintain our house in good shape to avoid decay, while we neglect to see a physician on a regular basis or disregard doctor's advice about eating habits and exercise.

It is only after years of consuming the wrong stuff that infirmities may become evident. Eat too much salt and you will develop hypertension, eat the wrong carbohydrates and you may get diabetes. Gout, once a disease of the rich, is making a comeback as a consequence of eating too much beef and seafood. Eat solely proteins and cardiac disease may ensue.

Old times, at least as far as eating patterns and the link to disease
were concerned, were the good old times. Food tasted better and did not make us sick.

The emergence of obesity and the spread of information about the condition have created a consensus to look carefully at what we eat, the composition of foods and how we cook them, and yet obesity is still a public hazard. As difficult as it is to tackle this problem, it is time for change.

We should refuse to eat hamburgers prepared with trimmings added to the ground beef because not infrequently they are contaminated with E. coli, sickening some and killing others (in the US alone there are 76 million cases of food-borne illnesses, as a result of which 5000 people die every year); or corn treated with insecticides and herbicides that have shown to produce organ failure in many experimental and clinical settings, or luscious desserts... and the list of the *forbidden fruits* goes on and on. We need to be serious and thoughtful when it comes to our eating practices. We have to regain the power to do what is right before we reach a point of no return.

Good nutrition is the first step to engineering our wellbeing. **You will be surprised to learn how one can achieve optimal health by eating the right things in the proper amount, like a specific group of fruits and vegetables which may help in becoming resistant to disease and even reverse existing medical conditions when combined with other steps.**

7

THE BASICS

In order to be the master of your destiny, at least when it comes to your health, you have to have certain knowledge. You may not know the principle of the internal combustion of the engine that moves your car but at least you understand that it will not run on an empty gas tank and that if something goes wrong, a light will flash on the dashboard and alert you that there is a malfunction. Unfortunately, when there is a slow disruption of your wellbeing there are no gadgets available to warn you that something is about to make you sick. When symptoms appear it may be too late to fix the problem. That is why is important to have periodic examinations in order to detect incoming or ongoing health issues. To have a minimal understanding of body functions is also a way to be alerted when there is a disruption.

When it comes to your health, knowledge will empower you to make the right decisions, and behave by your own design and do what is best for you. Once you are enlightened by the facts surrounding health issues you will be in command to use your brain and your emotions to do the right thing. You will discard false enticements, avoid the temptation of the allure created by food commercials and resist consuming noxious foodstuffs. Knowledge of health matters is bliss.

The more you comprehend the fundamentals of your body, the better you will be able to sieve the good from the bad when it comes to eating.

The first critical question is: how do we add unnecessary pounds to our body? The answer is simple and complicated at the same time. One would expect that, as with other automated bodily functions, our weight should remain within the parameters of what is considered normal. This is what the heart and our lungs do; for example, our heart beats 72 to 80 times a minute, give or take, when the body is in a resting state; the basal respiratory rate is 12 to 18 breaths per minute. The heart and the lungs adjust to compensate for our needs; for instance, exercising strenuously brings the breathing and the heart rate up, responding to the challenge of providing needed oxygen, and it does so in proportion to the amount of exertion up to certain limits. Longstanding physical performance brings the heart to beat at a slower rate in a resting state (let's say 46, instead of 72) because the heart becomes a more powerful pump, delivering as much oxygen in one beat, when before it delivered the same amount of blood in two.

The same happens with other body mechanisms. For example, our body temperature is about 97 degrees Fahrenheit with little up or down variation provided by a fine thermoregulatory mechanism. Infection, inflammation and other conditions will reset the temperature to a higher point. Specialized cells, called monocyte-macrophages, elaborate cytokines, which causes elevation of the thermal set point through a part of the brain called hypothalamus.

The capacity of our body to maintain function at stable levels is called homeostasis. All of this is done by a complex physical and chemical process. If it fails we get sick or die.

When it comes to weight regulation one would expect our wise human body, after eating more than we need, would shut off our appetite so we can eat less or at least provide some automatic function to burn extra calories. But this does not happen with everybody; there are some who have a relentless need to eat and the more they eat, the more weight they gain. This is not perplexing; our body is good to us providing we are good to it. It is interesting to note that when pets are not allowed to roam freely and are overfed they become obese, something not seen in wild animals, which eat only according to their needs, thus keeping their homeostatic mechanism intact.

This does not only happen with eating; there are many examples of abuse and physical failure: smokers lose their functional lung capacity because pulmonary damage alters its physiological response; cocaine addicts get heart damage, impaired function and cardiac insufficiency. In the same way overeating disrupts weight balance. These are three similar situations where a noxious agent produces a breakdown in function. Excessive food intake becomes toxic like tobacco, drugs and excessive alcohol and similarly leads to addiction.

Excess weight then should be viewed as an **injury** that triggers a malfunction of our superb homeostatic mechanism **altering the shape and function of every cell of our body.**

The two crucial components of weight are intake and output. Intake refers to the calories we eat and drink and output to how many calories we burn while performing our daily routine.

In order to maintain the normal function of our organs and to support our daily activity we need energy, which is supplied by what we eat. Food is fuel. The requirement for the average person is 1800 to 2000 calories a day. This figure is to be corrected for growth, pregnancy, age, sex, amount of physical activity and other variations.

Here is one **normal** departure: There is a 24 year old gentleman who eats 8,000 to 10,000 calories a day. His height is six-feet-four and he weighs 190 pounds. He is trim and athletic. His weight has remained stable, which means that his daily caloric expenditure has to be around 10,000 calories. For breakfast he eats fried egg sandwiches, for lunch and dinner, among other foodstuffs, a lot of pizza and pasta, and yet he is in good health. Did you guess who he is? Here are some clues. He is not a banker but makes as much money; he works shorter hours but harder and has won 14 Olympic medals. Your presumption is correct: he is Michael Phelps. He trains about five to six hours a day. Since with recreational swimming we burn up 500 calories an hour, Michael during training or competition may be kindling 1500 calories an hour. The intake of eight thousand calories in people with sedentary life will produce obesity and all kinds of infirmities, from a heart attack to cancer, to name a few.

Ontologically, the human and the animal body come well equipped for survival and preservation of the species. Hunger, thirst and sex drive are necessary to maintain and perpetuate life. The animal kingdom (humans included) possesses a perfect machine that is only made imperfect when we interfere with its function.

We get hungry because our alarm system tells us that it is time to replenish the needed energy provided by food. This energy is stored and used as needed to grow, move, fight disease, make love, think—essentially to live. Everything starts in the brain, specifically in the hypothalamus, a command center located behind the eyes. It controls a wide range of functions such as sexual behavior, hormone production and emotions, and commands the peripheral autonomic nervous system, which is responsible for all visceral functions like breathing, regulating heart rate, digestive function, and perspiration, among others. A myriad of systems are essential in regulating eating behavior. The hypothalamus (like every single cell in our body) constantly talks to every other organ. It interacts with the stomach, which releases ghrelin, a hormone that stimulates appetite. This initiates a cascade of events with metabolic consequences within the liver, the pancreas and the endocrine system. Ghrelin also is produced in the *arcuate nucleus* of the hypothalamus and plays, among other things, an important function in the learning process. After we eat enough, ghrelin tells the fat cells of our body to release another hormone, leptin, to give us a sensation of satiety so we can stop gorging. To make it more graphic: a newborn is irritable, restless, awakes from sleep; she is hungry; she just has released a substantial amount of ghrelin. After being fed by her mother satiety kicks in, leptin is released, she experiences a sensation of pleasure, her hyperirritability goes away and goes back to sleep. This repeats again in a cyclical fashion and assures that she will receive the right amount of nutrition for growth and development. This tantalizing machinery works perfectly within certain boundaries. Only interference by humans disrupts its fragile function. Eating more than needed at any stage of our life is the culprit in getting us out of balance, a disruption that is difficult to overcome.

At the beginning of the chapter we asked why there is a crack in the physiological mechanism that makes us fat. As we have seen, things should be uncomplicated. Match calories ingested with calories spent, problem solved, since nature, as we have seen, has provided us with precious, magical regulatory mechanisms to stay fit and healthy. Regarding a genetic factor which may predispose an individual to be fat (and we know very little about the role of genes and obesity), the answer has been sought by scientists for decades. Some had directed their research in trying to find a substance that might trigger people to eat too much, others have measured different hormonal levels of obese people and compared them to normal ones while still others have looked at brain function with the hope of discovering the missing piece of the puzzle.

The answer appears to be simpler, independent of the mechanism: We are fat because we eat too much or don't exercise enough. Many times we use food to calm our anxiety or overcome emotional distress; food acts like a pacifier and an antidepressant, so we overeat. The problem is compounded by environmental causes, resulting in a disruption of our normal physiology. Our lifestyle influences our health and sometimes is not shaped by our physical or emotional needs or inclinations but by the design of others. Food is more available and cheaper than ever before. The food industry wants us to eat more because the more we eat the larger their economic reward. They have the money and power to entice us to consume what they sell. Their marketing strategies are powerful and irresistible. It is the abundance and availability of soft drinks, prepackaged foods and harmful edibles that are everywhere, in food outlets, restaurants, and fast food eateries, that makes us sick, a nation of fat people where epidemiological studies unequivocally show an increased incidence of diabetes, cancer, arthritis, degenerative and inflammatory diseases, heart failure and hypertension.

8

Dietary recommendations:

Basic and simple information enables us to recognize which nutrients are detrimental and which are helpful in keeping us fit and healthy. **To be more emphatic, albeit repetitive: proteins and complex sugars are the desirable part of any diet; simple sugars and fats, especially saturated fats like the ones from animals, are unwelcome.** These concepts need to be entrenched in us to discern what is good and what is bad when it comes to choosing what we eat. The familiarity with nutrients will transform your eating habits, the same way that learning how to use an electronic gadget allows taking advantage of its features and maximizing its use. After a while, being on familiar terms with the content of food becomes second nature. You won't need to stop and consider if what you are about to eat is good or bad.

When we watch a football game with friends, drinking beer and munching all sorts of snacks like corn chips, dips, donuts, we are usually ingesting 1500 calories or more, which represents more than 2/3 of our daily nutritional requirements. Knowing the harm we are inflicting to our body, we may have the opportunity to think twice before eating them and replace them with cereals, fruits, vegetables and nuts, which are tasty and readily available.

Nutritional requirements vary from individual to individual depending on sex, age, body frame, height, associated medical conditions, and pregnancy. The energy needs are also dependent on daily activity. We mentioned before that Michael Phelps consumes about 10,000 calories a day when he is training and expends the same amount of energy, which explains how an overeater may be endowed with normal biological parameters. It is difficult to define an 'average person', yet for practical purposes we accept that 1800 to 2000 calories a day are needed for most of us to maintain a stable weight.

Calorie expenditure varies in different circumstances: sleeping 8 hours a day will burn about 560 calories; sitting for 8 hours, 800, housekeeping chores or shopping or walking for three hours, 600; moderate exercise for one hour, 300 hundred; and heavy workout, like playing any sport or swimming, about 600 calories. Half an hour of sexual intercourse burns about 200 calories.

The amount of calories that a person needs to consume varies according to the purpose of either maintaining weight or shedding pounds. To determine this, one needs to take into account a series of variants, like height and body frame, and make corrections according to daily activities. Establishing a target facilitates achieving a goal. Nutritionists, physicians, trainers, books or the Internet can provide needed information. A friend of mine, I will call her Laura, has a personal trainer and she works out very hard one hour a day five times a week. She started doing this to lose weight (she gained 25 pounds after pregnancy). A workout routine like hers should have produced excellent and measurable results, though it has been now three years and she remains as chubby. Laura is in the same predicament as millions of people who go to the gym routinely and who cannot shed pounds because they eat more than what they burn. Exercising so one can eat indiscriminately is the wrong approach, although better than not doing any physical activity at all.

9

The Ideal Diet: In western culture people have common aspirations, some in the material and others in the spiritual realm. We long for security, good education for us and our children and good health. We know that good health is linked to proper eating and yet we don't know exactly what this means or how to go about it. We read and hear that good food equates to being well and preventing diseases that are pervasive in our society and what appears to be a simple proposition—eating quality food, drinking the right stuff, both in the proper amount—is a sticky daily event. Unless one adheres to a planned routine that encompasses avoiding the wrong kind of edibles, one is bound to become, sooner or later, sick with an infirmity. This is an abstract concept, until a disease hits. Being and staying healthy is like the wish of many to make a lot of money but not knowing how to go about it. This simplistic comparison has certain parallels. In both cases people read guides, or self-help books, usually with little success.

What you will read next are uncomplicated truths, unpretentious and unadorned. We definitely know a great deal about the composition of foods, the extent of their worth and their influence on health and disease. In the past, scientific nutritional facts were only accessible to professionals, while today the knowledge is in the public arena for everybody to see and grasp.

The ideal diet is one that provides optimal nourishment and is palatable, accessible, affordable and easy to follow. Daily consumption of macronutrients should include 130 grams of carbohydrates, 35 grams of fiber, 50 grams of protein, no more than 30 percent of calories from fat, 3.7 liters of water for males and 2.7 for females, linoleic acid, omega-6 and omega-3 fatty acids and little or no cholesterol, trans fatty acids, saturated fatty acids, sugar and salt. Alcohol (preferably a moderate amount of red wine, with some exceptions), vitamins and minerals should be part of a normal diet. Since it is impractical to measure and make a distinction in our daily routine of how much we eat of each of these nutrients we need to develop a mechanical routine. **A sensible and realistic way to eat is to have the mindset to eat predominantly quality carbohydrates, a moderate amount of protein and as little fat as possible.**

This ideal diet contains enough of every element that may prevent cancer or fight disease, with a caveat: nutrition is an evolving and dynamic discipline, so what we believe is correct today may be wrong tomorrow, reflecting the constant search to find the right answers to difficult problems. Yet in this era there is enough information to be able to outline a no-nonsense and realistic diet that may prevent sickness or enhanced recovery from an illness.

Often patients who contract a fatal disease ask, "Why me? Why if I always ate the right thing and exercised five times a week?" These kinds of questions humble us because we don't have all the answers. But we have some, which is what this book is all about: describing the pillars that support our wellbeing and that can help in precluding or delaying the appearance of dreadful conditions. Knowledge is power.

Asbestos exposure is the cause of mesothelioma, a condition that affects the lungs and other organs and is invariably fatal; excessive mercury produces neurological defects; too much

Vitamin D may trigger heart problems, and the list of environmental poisons is endless. It follows that knowing this, should lead us to do the right thing to preclude their appearance. The same is true with environmental agents responsible for triggering serious medical conditions. The problem is that they are everywhere, pervasive, in the food we eat, the water we drink and the air we breathe.

Cancer and other ailments are multifaceted in their origin and behavior. Animal experimentation, clinical studies, analysis of epidemiological data, chemical investigations and laboratory studies are some of the methods scientists use to solve the quandary of disease. The theory is that a combination of an external factors (as mentioned above) hitting a predisposed terrain (us) triggers a disease; therefore by understanding both, noxious outer elements and our body, we may be able to exert some control in preventing disease.

The advances in medicine are tantalizing and thanks to them we have lengthen lifespan although not always the quality of life. Progress in the understanding of disease could be viewed as a pyramid formed by stones which have been laid at its base since time immemorial . Today we are still far away from the zenith; many more stones will need to be added, carefully and judiciously, with logic and wisdom, before we can claim success.

Dr. David Servan-Schreiber is a physician who had a brain tumor first diagnosed in 1994. At that time he and two other colleagues were investigating brain function in humans utilizing functional magnetic resonance imaging (MRI). They were looking at the variation in images at the level of the brain in individuals performing specific mental tasks designed to stimulate the organ at a maximum. On one fateful day, one student who was part of an experiment did not show up, so David was asked to volunteer and step into the scanner. The initial images showed that there was something wrong in his brain. This serendipitous finding was confirmed by the radiologist the next day: David had a malignant tumor. The cancer was removed, chemo and radiation therapy followed, only to have the cancer recur years later, necessitating another round of therapy. He decided to take things into his own hands and, without abandoning his conventional medical care, started to investigate other means of fighting his condition and avoiding a recurrence. He embarked on a special diet, started exercising on a regular basis and sought peace of mind by meditation and other means. He succeeded for sixteen years but later died from a recurrence, yet he survived much longer than expected for somebody with this condition. Dr. Servan-Schreiber felt compelled to share his experience in the book *Anti-cancer: A way of Life.* In one of the chapters he explains that angiogenesis, or the formation and proliferation of vessels observed in certain tumors, is the phenomenon that allows growth and spread of many cancers. This is facilitated by a chemical substance called angiogenin, which can be blocked by another chemical called angiostatin. Making angiostatin prevail causes tumors to regress or disappear. This concept led to the development of Avastin, a drug which mimics angiostatin and is partially effective in treating certain tumors, **and to the discovery that certain herbs, spices, green tea and edible mushrooms can block the effects of angiogenin**.

Inflammation is the common response of the body to any type of injury, internal or external, and is a precursor to cancer. Fighting inflammation may prevent its formation. Besides medications, many fruits and vegetables contain substances that are effective in controlling inflammation. Exercise and emotional balance, which we discuss in Chapters 5 and 6, also have a therapeutic effect in fighting disease.

During the last decades much knowledge has been acquired through science, but at the same time so little has passed from the research centers to the public.

Eating well is complicated and distressing since it is difficult to escape our cultural leanings. Later, we will discuss how to achieve dietary goals. The only way to be able to conform to a normal diet is to unravel the weight paradigm, disentangle the myths, denounce lies and deceptions, and adhere to a sensible plan. You will reach a point when suddenly eating well and the right amount becomes pleasurable and gratifying.

10

Before this, some comments about our urge to overeat, what we and others call an addiction. Whether overeating is a true addiction or a compulsion is still debatable; nevertheless, it needs to be differentiated from other dependencies like smoking, drugs and alcohol. These substances are not indispensable for survival and need to be set apart from excessive food intake. Food has calming effects, which is why many who are unable to achieve satisfaction in life seek solace in food. Addictions seldom disappear if the affected individual doesn't give them up completely. Alcoholics cannot have an occasional drink, smokers an occasional puff and drug addicts a once-in-a-while recreational drug, otherwise a recurrence would most surely occur. Perhaps it would be better to understand overeating as a bad habit or a craving to take away the stigma, the guilt and the shame that goes along with the word addiction. This will help to confront infatuation with food at a different level, take away the need to justify why you eat so much, and remove the stress associated with overeating and the humiliation of being overweight. Eating provides joy and comfort, tempers stress and calms anxiety, which explains in part our need to eat beyond our needs.

The problem of overeating is compounded by accessibility of edibles and by the lure that the food industry artfully creates to entice us to consume.

Whether overeating is simply a compulsion to eat or an addiction deserves one more paragraph. For the reader it may be a matter of semantics but for a scientist interested in health matters, it is a crucial question in order to guide any investigation. Compulsive behavior may be treated by antidepressants and behavior modification techniques, while addiction requires detoxification programs, group therapy, family involvement and behavior intervention. The matter is not settled yet, which in part explains why there is no definitive treatment for obesity.

The first step to embark on eating the right way is to recognize that you are free to choose what you eat without imposition from others; by understanding this, you may be able to discard the influence of the food industry which through marketing and advertisement tries to persuade and tempt us to consume their products.

You don't need to feel embarrassed or mortified because you are eating too much or the wrong stuff; with time you will be able to make the right decisions regarding amount and quality of food and understand that occasionally you can indulge in eating your favorite meal without creating havoc with your health. You will get physical and intellectual satisfaction when savoring a small cone of ice cream with 300 calories instead of the large one with 900 because it is your decision, because you are in control.

The habit of overeating creates a disruption in the brain circuit and a dysfunctional hormonal response that is reversible. The gratification of overeating can be replaced by the satisfaction of being the one that freely decides how much to eat.

A basic knowledge of nutrients will make it easy to adhere to a plan. Diets should not be strict; one should not obsess about eating habits and should understand that temporary treats may be compensated for at a later time by eating less. Today is Thanksgiving; Mother is preparing her usual turkey with all the hypercaloric trimmings, so be it, just eat it. Tomorrow you will eat a light meal to compensate and move on—no shame, and no guilt.

Crash diets do not work, appetite suppressants are useless, fad diet books are a waste of time and money, and the food gurus are worthless. Take your time; create the habit by the relentless pursuit and the deep understanding of what is good for you. In the end, to stay fit and healthy is a spiritual journey and you will find the best for you, identify your strengths and recognize your power to change things. If you can conquer your bad habits you will be able to resist other temptations and your best qualities as a human being will flourish.

A diet program should always be accompanied with exercise and stress reduction.

Too much salt, fat and sugar are the enemies. Fresh vegetables and fruits are your friends. These recommendations have a strong scientific foundation. Salt, for example, when reduced to three grams a day, is projected to reduce the annual number of new cases of coronary artery disease by 60,000 to 120,000; stroke by 32,000 to 66,000; and myocardial infarction by 54,000 to 99,000; and to reduce the annual number of deaths by 44,000 to 92,000. These are impressive numbers and should entice us to keep the salt shaker off the table.

Keep the animals out of the kitchen as much as you can. Eating beef or chicken every day increases exogenous cholesterol, so at a maximum one should not eat meat more than twice a week. Fish has omega oils and it is a good substitute for other types of meats.

Nutrition is a discipline that has positively evolved in these last four decades, providing a core of knowledge that has benefited sick patients by tailoring diets to their specific condition; diabetes is the prototypical example. Today dietary guidelines are used to preserve wellbeing, prevent and cure illness, prolong life and improve stamina.

Is there a perfect diet? Should we all be eating like the Japanese, the Italians or the vegetarians, since they live longer? In reality there is no one single healthy diet regime but a set of sound principles. Consuming the right stuff and managing calorie intake prevents disease and slows down the effects of age. The goal at all ages is to be well by eating well all the time.

Eating well is being well; controlling urges makes people physically and emotionally stronger.

The basic concepts outlined above should suffice to discern what is good and what is bad when it comes to eating, so simple and yet so difficult. It is the amount and the quality of the products we consume that makes all the difference. We are not only what we eat, we are what we think, how we behave and what we can achieve spiritually, which in the end will determine how healthy we will be. All this derives from the knowledge we acquire and what we do with it.

With knowledge we don't need fad diets because in the past they all have failed us. Eating judiciously has a tremendous impact on our wellbeing, brings happiness and comfort and assures a long life. When it comes to eating, what we need is a new mindset, a different framework.

The following premises are essential for you to be able to become the master of your eating habits:

- Read the Nutrition Facts on food labels, which describe calories, composition, preservatives, chemicals and added salt; then compare and choose.
- Avoid processed foods.
- Don't settle for foods that are not tasty. A healthy food does not have to be unsavory.
- Excess salt, fat and refined sugars are your enemies.
- Compensate tomorrow for today's overeating.
- Dressing and sauces are hypercaloric. Don't allow them to smother your plate but rather allow them to just give a taste to what you are eating. Ask for the dressing to be served on the side.

- Whole is holy (grains that is).
- Don't allow animals to be frequent visitors into your kitchen (beef, poultry that is)—no more than twice a week.
- The secret is in the variation of foodstuffs; if not, you will become bored and soon abandon a meal program that with ample variation may become appealing to your taste buds.
- Organic is better.
- Added chemicals and hormones are bad.
- Fresh vegetables in season cost less and are tastier than refrigerated ones and preserve all the nutrients.
- The fundamental part of a diet should consist of grains, fresh fruit and vegetables. One serving of them amounts to one cup, and 4 to 6 servings of fruit and vegetables is the recommended daily amount.
- Fresh veggies go over everything: pasta, pizza, salads and sauces. They add taste and flavor.
- Be practical; have pre-washed bags of salad greens and veggies in your refrigerator, to which you may add a hypocaloric dressing. They are tasty, healthy and fulfilling.
- When you feel hungry between your main meals, grab fruit or veggies.
- Fat-free, low fat and reduced fat are welcome in any type or shape.
- Eggs have 13 excellent nutrients; egg white is always fine and whole egg no more than twice a week.
- Empty calories (table sugar) are dumb.
- Fiber is good. Very good.
- An occasional glass of red wine is fine, but no more than two a day.
- Don't patronize all-you can-eat buffets.
- Avoid restaurants that serve succulent hypercaloric foods.
- Fast food joints are not for you and not for your children.

- Don't succumb to the temptations of bread and butter before they bring your meal in a restaurant. They will add calories, almost as much as an entree.
- Make your own list of edibles that you enjoy and are nutritionally sound and make them the basis of your diet. Others that you may enjoy, like eggs, chocolate and red wine, are admissible if used sparingly.
- Eat three times a day and have one or two occasional snacks, preferably in the form of fruit or vegetables.
- Eating good, organic and tasty food, variation in edibles, cooking creatively and consuming the right amount of food with enjoyment is the way to remain fit.

Fixed, fad, fancy, special, detoxification, anecdotal, solely protein, solely fat, solely carbohydrate and other ill-conceived diets do not work in the long run.

A nutritional eating program is easier than you think. You are empowered to make your food choices. Don't obsess about food or eating patterns; make them part of your lifestyle. Stress and depression will let you succumb to overeating because food is comforting and nurturing, but bear in mind that too much of anything can be hurtful. Treat stress and depression by other substantive and effective ways. Combining mindful eating with exercise and emotional balance is the pillar to sustain your well being.

Knowledge is the instrument that eradicates superstitions and myths from our daily life, which can harm by precluding us from doing the right thing.

CHAPTER 2

NUTRITION – PART 2

CLIMBING EVEREST

It does not matter how slow you go as long as you don't stop.
- Confucius

1

Mountaineers know how difficult it is to reach the crest of Mount Everest; the attempts have cost hundreds of lives, and there have been thousands of failures. There are many factors involved in the drama of climbing the tallest mountain on Earth. Success depends on age, fitness, ancillary equipment, choosing the best path and guides, interaction with the natives and money, among other things. It is one of the most difficult adventures that man can attempt. It may sound foolish to compare this endeavor with the effort to lose weight, but I would ask the reader to allow me to use the climbing of Everest as a metaphor. The struggle, the physical and emotional pain when trying to lose weight, is analogous. For the climbers reaching the peak of a mountain is magical and gives them an immeasurable exhilaration and a sense of vast accomplishment. It brings them the majesty of nature in its entire splendor. Its peak is the crossroad of air, water and soil, where nothing else exists, and forces them to retreat to the inner self, a place where one can temporarily forget about wickedness and misfortunes.

For those who attempt a weight reducing diet and are victorious, the emotions are similar. Why not? Only two percent of people who decide to start weight reduction diets are able to stay fit after one year, which points to the enormity of the task. This is an impressive figure because statistics show that Americans spend over 40 billion dollars a year on dieting and diet-related paraphernalia. On any given day, millions of people in the world are dieting.

Diego Armando Maradona is a case in point. Diego is the FIFA (International Soccer Federation) Player of the Century and the most gifted soccer player who ever lived. After he retired from playing at age 37 (a very late age by the sport standards), he gained considerable weight, going from 143 to 266 pounds. After different attempts to reduce weight he underwent a gastric bypass in Cartagena, Colombia. After the operation he was slim and fit. Four years later he is putting on weight again. Today he looks chunky at 260 pounds or more. This underscores that even drastic measures like surgery may not alone resolve the issue of obesity.

Another illustrious case that demonstrates the problems associated with losing weight is that of Oprah Winfrey, the beloved television personality. In 1992 she weighed 237 pounds, in 2001 she started a diet program and in 2005 her weight was 160 pounds. She looked glamorous, fit, healthy and beautiful. Her achievement made news all over the world. She was praised and admired for her efforts, made the cover of many popular magazines and became a role model for many who wanted to lose weight. Slowly she added pounds, became fat again and confessed that food was like a drug that she used for comfort and to ease stress. She wrote, "I don't have a weight problem, I have a self-care problem that manifests trough weight…I dare all of us give all the love and care we need to be healthy, to be well and to be whole." If Oprah, a person of strong will and vast resources, could not make her weight loss stick, what can we expect for the rest of us mere mortals?

In 1985 a new, ingenious method for weight control was devised by Drs. Lloyd and Mary Garren. It consisted of the placement of a gastric balloon in the stomach, which was inserted and inflated endoscopically. The principle was that the balloon, by occupying large part of the space of the stomach, would mimic eating a large meal, producing early satiety and as a result, the patient would eat less and lose weight. The procedure was approved by the FDA to be used not exceeding a three month period. In order to qualify for the procedure patients underwent an initial psychological evaluation and were advised to enroll in nutritional counseling and behavioral modification classes. The manufacturer of the balloon, American Edwards Laboratory, promoted the use of the device by inviting endoscopists to learn how to insert it. The assembly and the retrieval of the balloon were not easy, but after a while practice made it simple. I learned the technique in 1989, strictly applied the recommended criteria and inserted it in 50 patients. My experience was very disappointing. Patients would lose intestine after it inadvertently deflated, which in some cases produced bowel obstruction. A fatality was reported in one case. Thankfully, none of my patients had a complication during or after insertion and removal. The procedure was abandoned years later because it was deemed inefficient and unsafe. This is an example of the many inventions to lose weight leading to nowhere.

As with any enterprise like climbing a mountain, starting a new business or losing weight, careful planning is needed; starting with surveillance of the terrain. In the case of weight, terrain means facts associated with eating in terms of quality and amount, the possibility of burning calories by increasing physical activities and exploring the way that our emotional life may affect achieving the intended goal.

Overeating is an indulgence and not recognizing it when it becomes an addiction makes treatment difficult.

I stopped admonishing my patients about their weight because I learned that lecturing and reprimands do not work. During my early years as a physician I worked at the National

Institute of Health in Argentina. Patients' rooms accommodated two patients. At one time, the Director of the Department of Gastroenterology, Marcelo Royer, an outstanding and internationally known gastroenterologist, decided to lodge patients with stable alcoholic liver disease with others who were terminally ill. His intentions were good. He hoped that the stable one by witnessing the misery of dying of the other would stop drinking. At the same time they were lectured about the harmful effects of alcohol. It never worked. Across the street from the hospital there was a restaurant where we would occasionally have lunch. One day when we entered the place we saw one of those patients, who we had discharged earlier, savoring a dish of spaghetti and drinking a full bottle of wine. Royer's idea was well intentioned, albeit perhaps unethical, but it never accomplished its intended purpose.

Obesity is a complex condition. The compulsion to eat arises from learned habits, the environment, internal needs, personality traits, dependence and by the lack of knowledge. In the following sections we will explain how people become fat and how addiction to food develops.

2

When eating becomes toxic:

Let's start with the premise that too much of anything can be deadly. In the long run fatness, alcohol, drugs and tobacco kill. Other pleasurable things may harm if carried to the extreme. Sex is pleasurable but obsession with or excessive sex will invariably lead to social, emotional and mental problems. In spite of the nefarious consequences of abuse, addicts have a very hard time getting rid of their compulsory behavior. A distinction should be made between food (and sex) and other addictions since eating and sex are necessary for survival while drugs, alcohol or tobacco are extrinsic to human nature.

There are several aspects related to eating too much, and entire textbooks and medical articles have been written about the subject. David Kessler explains in one of the chapters of his book *The End of Overeating: Taking Control of the Insatiable American Appetite* the process by which we overeat. He tells of multiple animal experiments, which can be extrapolated to humans, that show that eating too much of what we like gives more incentive to eat beyond satiety; in other words, we go further than satisfying our appetite and when we do so, we enter into a deranged cycle.

Sugars, fats and salt are palatable because they provide consistency, aroma and texture to a meal and different concentrations and added flavors make them very desirable. In animal experiments it was possible to make them overeat beyond their caloric needs by offering, within a controlled environment, tasty mixtures of nutrients; which runs contrary to the observation that animals in general maintain a stable weight. Anthony Sclafani, a researcher from the University of Chicago, showed that rats eating supermarket food would double their weight compared to rats that were offered only chow pellets. That was an eye-opener because it showed that animals subjected to conditions that mimic our eating patterns have the same biological responses we do. Easy access to tasty food leads to abuse and is sufficient to promote weight gain.

The food industry has mastered the art of creating appetizing meals in order for us to succumb to the temptation to consume them. Coupled with marketing and relatively low prices, the incentive to eat beyond satiety becomes difficult to elude.

I used to patronize the first Cheesecake Factory restaurant in Beverly Hills, California, in the early 80s. The place was famous for their pastries and their twenty variations of cheesecakes. The restaurant was small but the portions of food were humongous. Their fried chicken, hamburgers and the rest of the menu were mouthwatering. The owner, David Overton, was a nice, amicable guy, markedly overweight and a gourmand, who was in the restaurant every day attending to his customers. At that time calories and obesity, with all their implications, were not recognized as a health issue. The Cheesecake Factory then became one of the most successful restaurant chains, valued in the billions of dollars, with more than 150 locations nationwide. These restaurants, like others that are in the predicament of offering large portions of hypercaloric food at reasonable prices, are launching pads for obesity.

Kessler added another factor to explain our overindulgence, the reward drive that dictates what we eat. "The drive for reward aggressively asserts dominance over the drive for balance. It is not our biological destiny to return to a set point," he writes.

The compulsion for eating is something that we observe again and again in our contemporaries. Go to a restaurant with friends and see how many of them will eat bread soaked in olive oil or spread with butter before they even order their meal. Look at your seat companion in the plane and see how fast the food disappears from his plate. Watch how many times some people return to the table at a buffet dinner. Availability, variety and cost drive people to eat more.

Eating is pleasurable because it triggers a cascade of physiological phenomena that start with the liberation of dopamine and end with the release of endorphins, natural substances similar to opiates that produce a sense of wellbeing. Dopamine is produced in the adrenals and several areas of the brain. It is a neurotransmitter and a neurohormone released by the hypothalamus. It is a precursor of adrenaline (from the famous adrenaline rush). It has multiple functions: voluntary movements (which explain the use of dopamine enhancers in Parkinson's disease), mood, attention, learning, sleep, learning, lactation, pain processing, and sociability and for the purpose of our discussion, **motivation and reward**. The theory is that dopamine is released by naturally rewarding activities such as eating and sex. Smoking or drugs like cocaine also increase dopamine in the brain. There is a question about the role of dopamine providing pleasure or being a mediator associated with desire and motivation. When we smell food and we are hungry, the anticipatory desire releases dopamine, and when there is a prediction error, as when we expect a rewarding outcome that never materializes, the dopamine neurons become functionally depressed. Dopamine assists us in the decision-making process. When I go to Buenos Aires, my hometown, memories from my infancy come back as soon as I step outside the airport, which makes me seek some of the gratifications I experienced while living there. I rush to go to Fredo, the ice cream parlor that sells the best sabayon ice cream in the world, or to Dora Restaurant, where the shrimp is fresh not frozen and prepared exquisitely, like in no other place. I buy shoes, because after all, there is no better leather than in Argentina. All this starts in my brain circuits, where dopamine is released and commands me to go. It is the **anticipation** to recreate, eat, consume, that dictates my behavior. As a result endorphins are released, I have like a flush of an internal 'home-made' heroin, and I am happy; in reality, it is my brain talking to my heart because actually, according to my American friends who are food connoisseurs, told me after visiting Buenos Aires that they like Haagen-Dazs ice cream better, as well as the shrimp from Santa Monica Seafood Market in Los Angeles. And the shoes... are uncomfortable.

As I mentioned, the second phase of eating relates to the release of endorphins (from endo: internal and orphin: morphine). Endorphin is an opioid-like substance produced by the pituitary gland and like opium produces a sense of wellbeing and pain relief. When we eat, the brain-gut axis is activated and the interplay between dopamine and endorphins takes place. The Appetite Control System (ACS) regulates how much we eat. It is a regulatory center, kind of an Air Traffic Control Tower, dictating our eating behavior and as with planes, if it fails we crash.

Trader's Joe Swiss Dark Chocolate contains sugar, hazelnuts, cocoa mass, cocoa butter, milk and cocoa powder. One 20 gm. square has 120 calories. It is an epicurean treat difficult to resist. It is not difficult to understand how chocolate enthusiasts make the ACS fail by disabling the set-point responsible to tell them to stop gobbling, and when this happens the eating behavior becomes messed up. The system is based on the same program of the reptilian brain (the brain stem, the oldest region in the evolving human brain, similar to today's reptiles) where hunger and satiety run automatically at the primitive level. This arrangement may fail in humans because the sequence eat - stop eating- does not seem to follow the logic of nature and as we will see, we pay a steep price when altering the laws of nature.

My encounter with a young patient about 40 years ago illustrates the complexities and the precision of the brain circuitry. Ernesto was a nine year old patient from a low socioeconomic status. His mother said that for the last several months he had been eating dirt. I was disconcerted and asked a second opinion from my colleague Luis Colombato. This patient appeared to have an obsessive compulsive disorder and yet his behavior was normal in all other respects. Luis looked at him, noticed he was thin and pale, and had a smooth tongue and brittle nails. He ordered some tests that showed an iron deficiency anemia. He was given iron tablets and within six weeks his compulsion ceased. Ernesto was affected with pica, a rare disorder that affects mainly children and pregnant women and is characterized by the compulsion to eat non-food or raw-food substances to compensate for what is missing in their diet, an uncommon situation in industrialized countries but not infrequent in poor ones. Colombato explained that some individuals with nutritional deficiencies have a compensatory neurological response accountable for this 'eating disorder' which in this case is nothing but an adaptative response of the body to get what it needs. This example illustrates the fine tuning of ACS.

A nutrient provides nourishment and keeps a human body healthy, but the same one in large quantities becomes **toxic** (not to be confused with poisonous or contaminated). Saturated fats, concentrated sugars and some processed foods are **toxic** when ingested routinely in large quantities. To be more graphic: French fries in deep fried trans-fat oil; corn chips, donuts and processed foods with added chemicals; sodas; etc. belong to this category and make us sick, albeit in the long run. In this context **toxic** means the ability of a nutrient to produce a failure in the ACS and as a consequence trigger organ failure. Excessive salt consumption, for instance, causes high blood pressure; too much sugar may trigger diabetes that may have been in a dormant state; foods with high concentrations of uric acid may produce gout, etc.

The Appetite Control System is sensitive, and moderate attacks will make it fail. Exposure to highly rewarding food and constant overeating triggers a breakdown of the system. The industrial food establishment is keenly aware of how to assail our instincts and has created thousands of edibles that are appealing although noxious in the long run. Since it is difficult to prove that certain foods are toxic, there is little that governmental agencies, like the Food and Drug Administration, can do to curtail their use. The most they can accomplish is to alert the public that excessive consumption may be harmful in the long run.

Kessler, in *The Business of Food: Creating Highly Rewarding Stimuli,* explains what goes into the preparation of what otherwise look like innocent dishes. For instance, in a restaurant the salad may look 'healthy' because of the lettuce but the dressing and other additives creates a rather hypercaloric stuff. His detective work took him to different restaurant chains and food processing plants, where he discovered that nothing is what is seems to be. Artificial ingredients are so well developed that it is hard to tell that they are not the real thing, which makes it difficult to tell a natural food from a processed one.

Food manufacturers, restaurant chains and their offshoots are giving us the illusion that what we consume is good for us; after all, if something tastes good, it has to be good. It is not. Peel the onion of the industrial food chain and no matter how it is disguised, we end up with the same: too much sugar, too much salt, and too much fat. Too much saturated fat leads to atherosclerosis, myocardial infarction, stroke, obesity and probably cancer of the prostate and breast. Too much salt causes hypertension and water retention. Too much sugar can cause diabetes with all it secondary ailments: heart, kidney, eye, peripheral vascular disease, etc.

High Fructose Corn Syrup (HFCS) today is of interest because of its role in triggering disease. We use to assume that canned tomato sauce is a combination of fresh tomatoes with a little bit of salt, oil and garlic; that breakfast bars contain optimal nutrients; that bread is flour and water; that preserved soups are cooked as mothers do; and that bottled orange juice is a healthy concoction. This is not the case because of the omnipresence of HCFS, chemicals, dyes, preservatives and flavor enhancement substances loaded with calories and toxins. Excessive calories also come from fat and proteins, but the availability and the ubiquitous presence of HCFS makes it the main culprit.

The food industry has mounted a campaign to defend the use of High Fructose Corn Syrup. On their TV commercials they claim that it is a sugar not different from others, with the same caloric value. While this is true, what they don't say is that it is the abundance of this sugar and its poor nutritional value that makes it unhealthy. Who would expect that yogurt would contain HFCS? Similarly, many other non–suspect, supposedly healthy foodstuffs, like cheese, canned fruits and vegetables, once they are processed and subjected to industrial manipulations, become contaminated with all kinds of undesirable ingredients.

Corn plantations use fertilizers and insecticides and sometimes the corn is cultivated on the same land year after year in lieu of other crops, and this causes soil erosion, posing a serious hazard to the fields. This adds an ecological dimension to the HFCS quandary.

The beverage industry supported a research study that showed that HCFS is similar to other sweeteners. The fact that high fructose corn syrup may be as good as table sugar does not negate the fact that table sugar is as bad as high fructose corn syrup, because neither have nutritional value. Sugars are best delivered by fresh fruits and vegetables, because they also contain vitamins, minerals and fiber.

Other common ingredients of processed foods are saturated or trans fats, which increase cholesterol and contain nine calories per gram, which is more than twice those provided by carbohydrates and proteins.

When it comes to fat, we need to make a distinction: unsaturated fats in moderation are good because they modestly decrease total cholesterol and low-density lipoprotein (the bad one). Omega-3 fatty acids are beneficial because they decrease the risk of heart disease and help in lowering blood pressure. Omega-6 fatty acids are good but only if they maintain a ratio of less than three to one with Omega-3, otherwise the excess may have a pernicious effect, producing multiple medical conditions by causing inflammation of arteries due to the high content of linoleic acid. However, a recent study by William S Harris from the University of South Dakota published in *Circulation: Journal of the American Heart Association* in February of 2009, showed that patients having 5-10% of their caloric intake a day from Omega-6 decrease their potential incidence of coronary artery disease by at least 24% when compared with a control group. Further studies will be needed to clarify this finding.

It is our lifestyle, where eating occupies center stage, and the lack of social and corporate responsibility that set off the habit of indulgence.

Since sixty percent of people are overweight, we need to understand why the other forty percent are not and have a normal body mass index. This is not an easy question to answer because it has multiple facets: biological, social, political and environmental.

These are some of the uncertainties:

Is the limbic system of those who are not obese unaffected from pernicious stimuli?

Are we at the mercy of the food industry, which incites us to eat more and more?

Are we free to decide what to eat when we are under stress, since food is like a medicine that provides comfort and ameliorates suffering?

Should we be judged if we get a one dollar cheeseburger because we don't have the resources to pay for a better meal?

Have fat people a different wiring in their brains brain, starting a cascade of pathophysiological events that are beyond their control?

There are more questions related to eating behavior; the answers are biological and existential.

We know more about abnormal behavior than we do about normality. Research is being conducted on people who have weight problems and seldom on normal individuals.

Gail Zweigenthal, a former editor of *Gourmet* magazine, is trim and slender. She says, "If I feel fat, I cannot enjoy eating." This may be true for those who are slim and healthy and get more satisfaction from their ability to control their desire to overeat and to stay in good health. My theory is that the dopamine mediated reward system may act not only by responding to sensorial stimuli derived from the physical act of eating but also by the intellectual gratification and emotional pleasure that one may get for exerting a strong will. In other words, we may get the same reward (endorphin or opioid-like substance release) if we overeat as when we make an effort to stop eating beyond satiety. When sensory or intellectual gratification is exaggerated it becomes pathological and as a consequence, we develop an eating disorder—obesity if we eat too much and bulimia if we eat too little.

When the delicate line between energy needs (food) and hedonics (too much food) is trespassed, overconsumption ensues.

What happened to the food industry? In Tale of Two Cities we talked about milk being directly provided by the cow, vegetables and fruits being only organic and fresh. That was 70 years ago. Little by little, habits changed. Milk became pasteurized, sold in glass bottles first and then in cartons; for centuries only salt, sugar and vinegar were used to preserve food; bread had to be eaten the day it was baked, otherwise it would become stale, bottled chocolate milk, a real treat, was just that—milk and chocolate. Then, with the need to transport edibles over long distances, preservatives were added. Competition among food manufacturers made them concoct products that looked better and were cheaper but not necessarily healthier. Strawberries became redder and much larger, hybrid fruits like the tangelo, aprium and about 50 others were introduced. Products containing sugar, salt and flour became prepackaged and had added chemicals. Wrapping became a thing of the past and was replaced by cans, plastic boxes and containers of all types. Fruits and vegetables are offered unripe to avoid spoilage. A long time ago fruits and vegetables were seasonal, with their nutrients intact. There was a joy brought by the expectation that seasons would bring: melons, strawberries and peaches in the spring; summer: grapes and mangos; winter: oranges and pears. The development of refrigeration and rapid forms of transportation ended the need for waiting but took away the bliss of anticipation and to make things worse, migratory fruits and vegetables lost flavor and aroma.

At one time, wines contained only small amounts of sulfites but later more were added to increase fermentation and avoid oxidation and spoilage; meats did not contain nitrites and nitrates, which still are considered carcinogenic by some; cheese, pickles, jams and a lot of other stuff were free of benzoates or sorbates and antimicrobial compounds.

Some fish are farm grown, sometimes as far away as Vietnam; they look like fish and taste like plastic.

Artificial ingredients are added to give texture, color, shape, form and aroma to what we eat. Rancidity is avoided by adding agents to slow oxidation of fats. Enzymes are added to delay ripening after harvest.

Food Packaging is part of a marketing strategy and edibles are now boxed up in fancy containers that may contain dangerous carcinogenic substances and paradoxically, the container usually costs more than its contents.

The same preservatives we found in household products like paint and medications can be found in the food we consume every day. Although BHA (butylated hydroxyanisole), a food preservative, and related compounds have been approved by the FDA, there are claims that they may produce cancer and behavioral problems. Dyes to give color to some of what we eat may produce bronchoconstriction, urticaria and angioedema, thyroid tumors, lymphomas and chromosomal damage, among numerous other ailments. Food additives used to make foods creamier or extend shelf life are safer in general, although some may produce allergies and headaches while others, like saccharin, are carcinogenic in animals, a fact that cannot conclusively be applied to humans. Sodium bicarbonate, which is used as a leavening agent and also to maintain acid balance in canned products, is a significant source of sodium, which is deleterious for those on a salt restricted diet.

Recently Suzy, a thirteen year old acquaintance of my family, was celebrating her birthday when suddenly, after she ate a shrimp appetizer, her face turned red and her voice became hoarse. A pediatric allergy specialist happened to be in the party and gave her an injection of epinephrine, which he carried in his doctor's bag. She recovered in a few minutes. Since Suzy had eaten shrimp many other times, it was the doctor's opinion that the allergic reaction was produced by some added artificial element like a dye or a preservative.

Pesticides, which are effective in preventing or destroying bugs, insects, vermin and mosquitoes, are used to protect plants, but are potentially toxic to humans. In the past DDT was a commonly used and highly effective insecticide in fighting malaria and other diseases transmitted by different vectors, but it was abandoned because it was linked to breast cancer and other ailments. Now DDT is only used illegally in underdeveloped countries.

Sulfites are potent allergens, mainly in children with asthma, and may cause swelling of the throat and hives.

The Environmental Protection Agency (EPA) is the regulatory organization in the United States that oversees the safety of the products we use or consume and is in charge of banning toxic carcinogenic or mutagenic substances. In spite of the oversight and regulations, from time to time, some approved products have to be recalled and removed from the shelves because they pose a health hazard. The American Medical Association has recommended limiting pesticide exposure and using those that are less toxic, advocating also the use of non-chemical alternatives like steam and other hot thermal interventions as disinfectants. It is known that agricultural workers exposed to chemicals have an increased incidence of health problems from neurological disorders, miscarriages and birth defects to cancer. Infants and children exposed to pesticide residuals in food are most vulnerable. New healthier alternatives have been developed to interfere with insect breeding, including genetic engineering, changes in cultivation practices or spraying plantations with hot water instead of chemicals. Antibiotics are extensively used in animals to prevent and treat disease; they act locally in the intestine and are not absorbed and therefore not passed to humans but their indiscriminate use is giving rise to new strains of bacteria with stronger resistance.

Hormones were at one time used in animals to promote growth and to increase the production of milk. Animals growing faster are slaughtered earlier, thus saving money by reducing waiting times and feeds. Their use today is illegal in the United States, because synthetic hormones passed to human increase cancer risk. Some food additives, although not hormonal by themselves, have estrogenic effects through metabolic conversion and therefore are potentially harmful. There are about 3,000 preservatives, flavorings, colors and other ingredients added to food produced by an innovative industry. Additives are used for other purposes beyond preservation; for instance, 4-hexyl resorcinol prevents discoloring of shrimp, lobster and other shellfish, while 4-Propyl gallate prevents fats and oil from spoiling.

Genetic engineering (GE) is a technique that changes the DNA, the carrier of genetic information, of living organisms. Scientists can split, manipulate and insert modified genes into a living organism for multiple purposes. In the early 1990s an insect-borne virus threatened to ruin Hawaii's papaya crop. A group of scientists isolated and copied one of the virus genes, which was then injected into the cells of the papaya plant, which made the fruit resistant to the virus. GE also makes crops stable, grow faster, pest resistant; it makes fruits more palatable, increases the amount of vitamin content and makes some bacteria a source of enzymes that can be used to process food. But GE is not as safe as we may believe.

There is public concern that genetic manipulation creates genetic pollution by uncontrolled spread and interbreeding between natural organisms. Greenpeace stated that "...biological diversity must be protected and respected as the global heritage of humankind, and one of our world's fundamental keys to survival... when we force life forms on our world's food supply to conform to human economic model rather than their natural ones, we do so at our own peril..."

Although there is no labeling required for genetically engineered products, sometimes it is easy to tell which foods are the end product of those manipulations, like the giant shiny strawberries, large peaches, contorted fruits or funny looking corn. Some genetically engineered foods have sacrificed taste for looks. Proponents of GE processing claim that this biotechnology decreases cost and sustains safety and availability of food around the world. Corporations don't want to see their profitability diminished so they oppose mandatory disclosure of processed food technology and are quick to dismiss social and environmental concerns. Some countries have imposed a ban or a moratorium on many food manipulations and added chemicals, out of fear that they may prove to be a long term health risk.

There was a profound transformation in the supply and manufacturing of food when corporations became the predominant provider. The path from nature to our table was once a single and simple phase, from the farm to our kitchen. Now the food industry is the purveyor of edibles of all kinds. They process, manufacture, distribute, market and sell most of the foodstuffs we eat.

Dr. John B. Phagan reported that in 1988 the Japanese company Showa Denko sold tryptophan produced in genetically engineered bacteria without safety testing because they and other companies had been selling innocuous non-genetically engineered tryptophan for years and considered that the two were biologically indistinguishable. Within few months it caused the deaths of 37 people and 1500 became permanently disabled. This underscores two important facts: a GE substance similar to its natural counterpart may be deadly and the safety of industrialized foodstuff cannot be taken for granted.

Adam Voiland, a Science and Medicine writer for *US News and World Report*, quoted a report from the Federal Trade Commission revealing that junk food makers spend some $1.6 billion annually advertising their products, while the *Journal of Public Health Policy* put the amount in the $10 billion range. The impact of these commercials has a serious public health impact. It is difficult to resist the temptation to eat a hamburger that is nicely presented on television commercials. Yet combined with fries and a large soft drink, they contain almost the total allotted daily amount of calories and large amounts of salt, sugar and fat.

Looking for sound advice regarding dietary recommendations is not easy; the food industry donates large sums of money to the American Dietetic Association and other institutions and this creates a conflict of interest that makes these organizations suspect of acquiescing to the industry demands.

Scientific jargon is frequently used in the discussion of the nutritional value of food and this confuses more than helps the consumer. The labeling on the packages may be purposely misleading, as well. For instance, a label asserting that a brand of yogurt is fat free does not mean that is low in calories, an intuitive conclusion. Yogurt contains about 100 calories per container, not a modest amount. Usually calories are disclosed per serving units, which are very small. For instance, a prepackaged pizza may disclose that it contains 450 calories per serving, so if we don't realize that this refers to one portion and eat the entire pizza, we end up consuming 1800 calories in one setting.

When it comes to safety, the food industry takes a cynical approach or manipulates existing information. It is frightening to observe the impunity with which they carry the slow, relentless spread of their products, which have no nutritional value or are harmful. They have mastered marketing to a point where the most attentive, watchful person may not resist the temptation of falling for what they sell; for instance, the food industry has now requested the FDA to change the name of High Fructose Corn Syrup to Corn Sugar as a way to disguise its bad reputation; labeling products with names like Power, High Performance, Energy, Nutri or the like creates the illusion of goodness; celebrities endorsing foodstuff incentivizes people to consume; funding of consumer groups artificially formed to promote a manufactured edible mask the real purpose of their support.

If what we just discussed is frightening, keep reading because the beast has not yet left the cage.

4

How civilized is the American Diet? Christopher Columbus changed the agricultural landscape of America forever by planting the first sugarcane roots that he took to Spain from what is now the Dominican Republic. America proved to be fertile and generous. To provide the manpower needed to cultivate the soil they brought slaves from Africa. Sugar was called white gold; at that time sugar was a very valuable commodity and was sold in pharmacies by the gram; when it appeared in Europe it created new industries and initiated a trend followed by coffee, fruits, chocolate, corn and other goods.

To this day the overplanting of crops without consideration to the long term effects has nefarious consequences, draining and exhausting the plains, depleting soil humus and devastating lands that once were lush and productive, converting some of them into a desert of rocks and weeds.

The agricultural transformation evolved slowly and the need to combat infestation, avoid spoilage and transport foodstuff produced at distant destinations changed the ecological topography, while at the same time it created new industrial and commercialization models. The linkage of bringing food from the field to our kitchen was simple, while now new constructs have created whole new methods, some good and some bad.

I first arrived in New York from Buenos Aires when I was 23 years old. I had signed a contract to start a rotating Internship at the Washington Hospital Center in Washington, D.C. I had never been in the States and for a young guy it was the adventure of a lifetime. My only contacts were Rosie, my grandmother's sister, and her three children, who I had never met before. They dined me and wined me; they showed me the lights of the city; and before I departed they presented me with their "old" five year old Ford, which was their spare car! My relatives were not rich and their gesture made me recognize the value of American solidarity, kindness and the regard they had for others. This is how my love affair with the United States started. New York was a gleaming and shining city; Brooklyn was a peculiar neighborhood. People were kind and willing to endure my poor command of the English language. A few days later I drove from New York to Washington on the New Jersey Turnpike (for me highways were one of the Seven Wonders of the World) to start my hospital assignment. On the way, I stopped in a fast food restaurant and ordered an archetypal American meal: fried chicken with fries, onion rings, strawberry pie and a Coke. This was my first encounter with the cherished American cuisine. One does not count calories at age 23, besides at that time, oil was oil, and sugar was sugar, with no specificity or qualifications. What I remember is that the meal tasted great, it was different from everything I had eaten before, I wanted more, and it helped me to start the ritual of honoring the beloved, tasty cookery of my adopted country. It is also true that as an intern I was making $200 dollars a month and could not afford to go to more sophisticated eateries. It was either eat in the hospital's cafeteria or at reasonably priced joints. Who would have said that years later I would abandon my passion and my delight for what once was the foundation of my appetite. It is not easy to ditch a first love, but my medical leanings prevailed over my instincts. It was seeing hundred of patients affected with ills produced by the harmful effects of civilization that alerted doctors that the population as a whole was eating too much of the wrong thing.

As a young physician I was puzzled by the allocation of disease. Why did Joanne, a 36 year old patient, mother of eight children, who had ulcerative colitis for six years develop fulminant colon cancer, a known complication of the disease, while Stewart, who had this condition for more than 25 years, was almost-symptom free? In medicine we have many unanswered questions. Among the possible theories to explain the etiology of certain conditions, we always entertained the idea that perhaps the lack or excess of certain nutrients may play a role in precipitating a disease. In some cases, like beri beri (deficit of vitamin B) or scurvy (lack of vitamin C), to name only two of hundreds of illnesses, the cause-effect relationship is proven, but the origins of many chronic diseases are still unknown.

This brings us back to corn:

Corn is a good, venerated food and one of the more resourceful plants on earth. As we mentioned, from corn we get our cooking oil, sugar, syrup, distilled spirits, alcohol, starch, high fructose syrup (HFCS), dry-process food, margarine, salad oil and flour. Today, most of the corn goes to feed livestock, which is then passed to us when we consume their meat or byproducts. In addition corn or the cob is used to produce nylon, plastics, paints, soaps, linoleum and gasoline, to name a few of its applications. The deserved respect for corn became dented by the misuse of the plant on several fronts. For one, it is present in most of the processed foods and its excessive consumption has dire consequences. Michael Pollan in his article *We are what we eat* informs us that the Big Mac patty and the chicken nugget contains 30 ingredients out of 37 made directly or indirectly from corn; French fries are fried in corn oil, salads composed of tomato and lettuce and sodas are mixed with sweeteners containing corn.

He writes, "If you are what you eat, and especially if you eat industrial food, as 99 percent of Americans do, what you are is corn," an impressive statement with multiple health connotations. Corn as an ever-present element, when processed, industrialized and used indiscriminately, initiates a cascade of infirmities, from obesity to diabetes to heart attacks, from its aggregated effect.

Corn is subsidized by the federal government, which explains its overproduction, which in turn leads to overconsumption. Salad dressings, yogurt, pastries, soups, packed or canned foods, sauces, certain breads and a very large part of supermarket foods contain this sugar.

In addition, food experts have determined that alpha amylase and glucose-isomerase, two of the enzymes used in the process of manufacturing HCFS, are genetically modified to make them more stable, extending the life of processed foods, and since it is cheaper than sugar it is been used more extensively. The availability and palatability induces **excessive intake,** which has been shown to impair growth and development in children. It is detrimental on two fronts, one by its lack of any intrinsic nutritional value and the other by replacing quality calories like the ones of sugar from cane or beets.

Dr. David Wallinga, Director of the Food and Health Program at the Institute for Agriculture and Trade Policy, reported that fifty percent of 55 tested retail products containing corn syrup are contaminated with mercury, a heavy metal that is neurotoxic, produces heart and kidney damage and compromises the immune system, a fact disputed by the Corn Refiners Association. Before Joseph Biden became vice-president of the US he was interviewed by Bill Maher, the political satirist, who asked him point-blank what kills more Americans, terrorism or HFCS. Unambiguously he responded, without minimizing the threat of terrorism, that HFCS is lethal and shortens the life span.

The battle between the merits and the disadvantage of corn syrup is escalating. Books, movies and articles in magazines, newspapers and the Internet are taking one side or the other. Today there is a public perception that High Fructose Corn Syrup is injurious. Responding to this, PepsiCo is now using cane and beet sugar in Pepsi Natural, Pepsi Throwback and Mountain Dew Throwback. Pizza Hut, Snapple and Kraft foods and ConAgra are also switching to natural sugars.

This is good and hopefully a trend to be imitated by the rest of the food industry, although it would be a mistake to forget that edibles containing a better sugar still deliver a large amount of calories. Dr. Pepper contains 150 calories, Schweppes Bitter Lemon 165. When **we exceed** our needed requirement by **300 calories a day,** we add weight. Obesity, dislipidemia, coronary heart disease, stroke, hypertension and type 2 Diabetes are the consequences of high consumption of HFCS (or sugar, for that matter).

Eating the wrong stuff has social implications, since we are all paying for the overeaters when they become sick.

The prevalent American diet is indeed **harmful**, not only from the excessive use of HFCS but also from the consumption of processed food and edibles contaminated with chemicals of all types. Luckily there is progress: the population is becoming more enlightened about the dangers of eating the wrong stuff; physicians, NGOs and GOs, celebrities, journalists, writers, and scientists are placing the problem on the front burner. In New York, for example, there is an ordinance for restaurants to list the amount of calories from each meal they serve, a small step in the right direction; ABC has a reality show called *Jamie Oliver's Food Revolution,* which aims to reveal the perils of overeating; the show is based in Huntington, a West Virginia city described as the most obese city in America.

The most hopeful fact to change the status quo is the passage of the Health Care Reform bill which contains provisions to put emphasis on prevention. There is universal recognition that eating healthy foods, promoting peace of mind and encouraging people to exercise may provide lasting wellbeing. Building a healthy life starts the day we are born.

The answer to the question how civilized is the American diet is simple: Not very.

5

Why are we in this predicament? We are what we know and what we do with our knowledge and the way we behave, which has individual and collective consequences, like our eating habits that are conducive to all kinds of ailments and now have become a national problem.

We have explained previously that our brain circuitry adapts to external stimuli and responds by releasing components that are set to maintain homeostasis. When the state of equilibrium becomes chronically impaired, we get sick. When our metabolism, which is the sum of the regulation of cell function, hormonal balance and fluid composition, among other complex activities, is attacked, it becomes deranged and we become sick. Eating too much sugar may bring diabetes, excessive drinking leads to liver cirrhosis, cocaine causes the heart to enlarge and fail, to give a few examples of what the constant intake of a noxious agent can do. When one organ becomes sick, the rest of the body becomes deranged because every cell in our body is interconnected. Hepatic cirrhosis not only affects the liver but also the anatomy and function of the esophagus (for instance by the development of esophageal varices that can bleed and kill a person), stomach, brain, skin and other tissues.

Chemicals, preservatives, genetic manipulation, additives, cultivation patterns and animal feeding practices involved in the industrialization of food have created a new genre of edibles unrecognizable from old, simple and traditional ones. As a consequence, the culture of eating has changed for the worse.

Not too long ago I experienced an inner moment of disconcertion. An acquaintance of mine brought his two and a half year old son to a meeting. The boy had long, curly hair; he was cute and adorable. I had an ephemeral love for the kid, augmented by the joy of anticipation because my daughter-in-law was pregnant. That same day during breakfast, I was reading the New York Times. One article was about the devastation that a bomb that failed to detonate would have caused in New York City; another about chemicals and cancer which, among other things, stated that "only a few hundred of the more than 80,000 chemicals in use in the United States have been tasted for safety...many known or suspected carcinogens are completely unregulated." As is usually the case, reading about dark and dismal events, makes me like everybody else, gloomy and sad, but as usual I moved on and continue to be the cheerful guy that I am, until I met Niko, the handsome kid. My fleeting moment of love was then followed by a preoccupation with what the future may bring him, my incoming grandchild and millions of others, in this world of ugly moments, hideous acts and horrible deeds.

As much as I am concerned by all this, I am more directly concerned with what I see and live and have lived every day of my life—the fact that there are a horde of silent killers out there. In medical school we are taught that hypertension is the *silent killer* since one may have the disease for decades without knowing it until one day it strikes in the form of a stroke or a heart attack. Later, I realized that other noiseless predators are taking charge of our lives and maiming us little by little. It may sound like an exaggeration to say that the deeds of many corporations have threatened and are threatening our well being, but is it? Asbestos has been known to produce mesothelioma, an invariably fatal disease, and yet it took years after this fact was well known to stop its use. Many medications—more about this later—have been withdrawn from the market, but not before killing thousands. How is it that we allow the food industry to maim us and no forceful reaction for change is taking place? For one, the damage is in the future and the future is an abstraction. Eating a lot of fat today won't do anything to an individual; eating the same amount day by day will kill him. Second, the recipients of the damage are anonymous; if the damage is done in one identifiable individual it would be different, but paradoxically since the injury is inflicted to many, we don't notice or we don't care. The food industry is good at switching the blame. They say it is not the givers but the takers that forfeit their individual responsibility, who abuse consumption of what in moderation would not hurt them.

The power of the food industry (which goes from the manufacturer to the provider) is enabling our poor eating habits. In the past we have succumbed to the influence of the tobacco corporations. The tobacco industry promoted smoking as a sign of masculinity, as when they created the Marlboro man; then in order to lure women they crafted a slim cigarette, a sign of glamour; commercials depicted ladies who smoked, fashionable, charming and seductive. Marketing was so successful that the tobacco industry became one of the richest manufacturing businesses in the world. The damage caused by nicotine is well known. Society took notice and governmental and private institutions mounted campaigns to discourage smoking. Taxes on tobacco were increased, marketing was curtailed, movies were not allowed to show casual smoking, cigarettes could not be sold near schools or playgrounds, the ill effects of nicotine were made public, and billboards announcing minute by minute the amount of deaths caused by tobacco made an impact in making people think twice before lighting a cigarette. The American Medical, the American Cancer and the American Heart Associations, to name a few, engaged in proactive campaigns to deter the use of tobacco. At local levels, counties and cities made smoking in public places a thing of the past, and as a result the consumption of cigarettes has come down from 631.5 billion a year to 360 billion. When it was recognized that passive smoking was harmful, it became a public concern, which prompted the passage of legislation to contain exposure to smoke.

Although late in the game, the consequences of eating the wrong stuff are a subject beginning to be tackled in the same way tobacco was.

Dr. Kessler visited many restaurants and interviewed more than 160 people for his book *The End of Overeating*. He talked with physicians, epidemiologists, nutritionists, psychologists, pharmacologists, neuroscientists, actors, chefs, addiction specialists, food experts, and weight loss consultants, among others, and revealed the practices of the food industry.

During his visits he uncovered the secrets that restaurants use to make food palatable. He learned how handling and combining different ingredients, use of additives, processing of food, plate presentation, and other techniques make their offerings difficult to resist. Food manipulations make popular restaurants like Chili's very successful. A company, Cinnabon, created cinnamon rolls that contained syrup, salt, sugar, caramel flavoring and other ingredients that make them irresistible. Pink's, a hot dog and Mexican food joint in Los Angeles, is patronized daily by thousands. I visited them some time ago. Having seen long lines of people day and night enticed me to go. I was curious to learn why the place is so popular. I ordered their staple, a hot dog and fries. I was not impressed; I had eaten better and worse. It is the power of our imagination that perpetuates myths and routines. The cost of my plate was 3 dollars and 50 cents, for that price I consumed 1100 calories in 15 minutes. This joint is legendary and has kept its appeal for more than 71 years.

Dr. Kessler describes how hyperpalatable foods came to be after he visited a Japanese restaurant in Manhattan and observed how shrimp was cooked "rolled in mayonnaise, fried in sweetened tempura batter, then rolled again in spicy mayonnaise," concluding "...that's fat on sugar on fat on fat." He went to Chinois restaurant in Santa Monica, Wolfgang Puck's famous chef eatery, where he observed how sizzling calamari salad was prepared in deep-fried rice oil, what he depicted as "...fat with a little lettuce." Antonio's Pizza, McDonald's, Grand Luxe Café, and a myriad of other restaurants were scrutinized. He discovered that their food is crafted with "...fat on sugar on fat on sugar on sugar."

He explained how fat helps flavors merge and has lubricating properties. Salt is part of the ingredients in sweet cookies and is also used in many unsuspected meals to make them appetizing.

The food industry has created, designed and commercialized food in such a way that we eat not what we need but rather what they want us to eat. Caution is required; not everything we eat is what we think it is. Who would have said that ice cream or meat may contain corn, or salad dressings may be stuffed with sugar? Who would have said that some vanilla ice cream has no vanilla and that orange drinks contain no oranges?

The fast food industry has an enormous influence in shaping our taste. They entice kids to consume chicken nuggets, nachos with copious melting cheese, and other hypercaloric items of little nutritional value. Burgers start at 99 cents (50 cents on Tuesdays), which makes them accessible to almost everybody. Coke, Pepsi or lemonade (manufactured without lemons) is now available in 12, 16 or 24 oz. cups that deliver up to 450 calories in a few gulps. If this were not enough, as Eric Schlosser writes in his book *Fast Food Nation: The Dark side of the All-American Meal,* fast food chains have formed partnerships with toy companies, sports organizations and Hollywood studios to attract kids, not by appealing to their appetite needs but to their inclination to play. Toys as a reward associated with a meal is a Pavlovian experience.

Does the food industry have a blatant disregard for people's health?

We are at the mercy of an organized structure that is interested in selling their products regardless of the nutritional value or it ill effects. This has a lasting and profound effect on our dietary habits. For their TV commercials they use photographs not of real food but rather a mixture of ingredients manipulated by digital equipment, lights, computers and props, making them irresistible.

The food industry may not see this as a problem; after all, a cheeseburger with fries and a soft drink does not kill anybody...in the short run. They don't recognize or don't want to acknowledge that the aggregate effect of poor quality food is harmful and in the end lethal. A parallel example is the impact that environmental pollutants have on our wellbeing. We are breathing contaminated air every day, but it takes decades to experience its consequences.

For most people, the fact that processed food may be toxic is an intangible concept. For us physicians it is not, because we see the devastation caused by obesity and other ailments with its consequences.

Perhaps the CEOs of the food industry may have a change of heart if they become in contact with patients, like Wendell Potter did. He was a CEO with Cigna, one of the largest health insurance organizations. He told Bill Moyers, the acclaimed television journalist, that while visiting his hometown in Tennessee he read in the newspaper about a Health Fair called Medical Expedition in Wise, Virginia. Out of curiosity he went to see it what all was about. It was a foggy day. There was a large open tent taking care of indigent patients who had come from South Carolina, Kentucky, Georgia and other nearby places. Volunteer dentists, nurses, physicians and veterinarians were providing care for thousands of patients (including cats and dogs) who could not pay. He had an epiphany and realized after more than 20 years in the health insurance industry that something was wrong with the system. Cigna was shifting costs from employers and insurers to individuals. The end result was that many people could not afford their premiums and so he realized that the practices of insurance companies were more about making profits than making sure that their enrollees were assured of having proper coverage; like those who could not obtain an adequate policy if they had a preexisting condition; others, after reaching a set cost, were left uninsured; while others after certain age could not be insured under the umbrella of a family policy, even if they were still living in the household with parents, or going to school and had no job. Seeing so many people in those conditions outraged Mr. Potter. It was like a lightning bolt. "I was insulated. I didn't really see what was going on. I saw the data. I knew that 47 million people were uninsured, but I didn't put faces with that number," he said. He quoted Dante who wrote, "The hottest places in hell are reserved for those who, in times of moral crisis, maintain neutrality."

I am drawing this parallel with the hope that food executives responsible for the slow maiming of people's health could walk the same path, become enlightened and take the same moral course. They are not the only villains of this story, however. Others include dogmatic nutritionists who preach the gospel of a diet without consideration to social and cultural values; doctors who concoct ingenious, appealing fad diets; the sellers of 'nutritional' supplements; the media that publishes articles about miracle diets without scrutiny; the marketeers at the service of the food industry devising misleading commercials; the parents who find it easier to substitute food for the love and emotional attention that their kids require; the professionals and non-professionals who take ownership of unfounded dietary recommendations and finally ourselves, who halt individual responsibility by allowing our hedonic impulses to prevail.

More than lifestyle modification, we need a profound cultural transformation that would arise from the understanding that in the long run we all may benefit from a profound change. Together we can become a nation of wholesome people; it takes commitment and dedication. We can do it.

Michael Pollan writes, "Food is also about pleasure, about community, about family and spirituality, about our relationship to the natural world, and about expressing our identity. As long as humans have been taking meals together, eating has been as much about culture as it has been about biology."

This is precisely the point: we can eat well, make the daily experience of eating enjoyable and use our common sense to stay fit and at the same time confront reality in a different way. It is through knowing and by exerting our will that we can be proactive and bring to ourselves permanent wellbeing.

There is another aspect that influences our eating habits, and that is our emotional life. In medical school or during training doctors are never taught how emotions, culture and other intangible social or personal issues may influence the health of individuals. Doctors are educated in a system that does not take into account patients' life situations. The curriculum in our universities is a restricted construct that does not include the personal life of patients as a variable, which as we now know, if left unattended prevents managing medical conditions with success. All this came as an awakening, when soon after graduation I was treating patients from different ethnicities who required different approaches to management, and patients with life stories that were influencing what we called the natural course of a disease. The power of positive thinking, faith, meditation and belief were ignored in the curriculum of most medical schools, thus preventing a useful complement to conventional medicine. It is the goodness of science combined with the understanding of other apparently insubstantial aspects of life that leads to a comprehensive management of the disease. **The definition of disease as a disorder**

caused by a known or unknown external element should be better defined as a disorder caused by internal or external elements that alters the physical and emotional stability of an individual.

In clinical practice we did not pay too much attention to the patient as a person because we were rigorously abiding by the rules we were taught in medical school, basically: diagnose with the tools of our trade and treat according to strict pharmacological criteria. The patient's lifestyle, stress, emotional life and social circumstances were ignored. Diabetes was treated with insulin, heart attacks with digitalis, hypertension with diuretics, with complete disregard to other factors. It takes a few minutes to take the blood pressure and write a prescription, while it takes a long time to interact with patients at a personal level, learn about their life, their family, counsel them about smoking cessation and nutrition, and yet it is in that realm that we can really cure instead of managing a disease. To make an impact we doctors have to learn new disciplines seldom included in the curriculum of medical school, namely, doctor-patient relationship, prevention, alternative medicine, belief systems, and the relationship between mind and body and the impact of lifestyle modification on health.

Before I jump to my final advice about how to eat well—in other words, how to climb the nutritional Everest—I need you to read the next chapter.

Chapter 3

NUTRITION – PART 3

Truths, Myths and Deceptions

Myths and creeds are heroic struggles to comprehend the truth in the world.- Ansel Adams

1

There is a necessary world of fantasy out there.

Some fantasies sustain our aspirations and creativity; others buttress our anxieties. It is there where the angels and demons live; they can save or kill us. In this world of fantasy we can find solace and renewal, stimulate our senses, and reawaken our dormant vices or virtues.

There is one part of this whimsical world that when brought to real life becomes a falsehood and when it relates to health may become a dangerous instrument.

It is remarkable to observe how people fall for myths and lies that promise good health, and yet it is also easy to explain: they fulfill a need for feeling safe and eternally young. Who wouldn't want to take a pill every morning to improve their stamina, another to make joints more flexible, one to increase sexual potency, and yet one more to make wrinkles disappear? Or follow the advice of a book that promises to make us slender and vigorous in five easy steps, books that are useless and after a while end up collecting dust. We all worry about our health and take different paths to calm those concerns; an easy way out is to submit to easy solutions.

Magic pills exist only in the imagination of others, who are pocketing billions of dollars from gullible people. Just pick up the newspaper, magazines or your local free weekly journal and you will see how many scammers are waiting for their prey. Google the word obesity or back pain or any other health issue on your computer and you will find thousands of bogus promises to solve those problems.

Infomercials and self-proclaimed health gurus have mastered the techniques of deception. The presence of so many books on subjects of health attests to the fact that there is an unfulfilled niche, cleverly exploited by many. The "last book you will ever need" is never the last.

Some cross ethical boundaries by promising cures for cancer where none exist and making patients forfeit the help they need. I recall many patients who out of desperation sought magical cures that gave them a ray of hope and ended up compounding their suffering and anguish. Jorge was a 45 year old patient of mine, a heavy smoker, who developed an aggressive cancer of the pancreas. When I first saw him the tumor had already invaded adjacent structures and metastasized to the liver. He was treated with conventional treatment, including radiation and chemotherapy, with poor results. He would not accept the seriousness of his condition. One day he came back to my office claiming that he was cured and was feeling a lot better. He had gone to a 'healer' in San Diego, who removed the cancer in a thirty minute session by 'extracting the cancer from his belly,' which he described as a piece of meat; when I asked him to show him the abdominal scar he told me that it healed within minutes and no residual scar was left. He died two days later. This case underscores the power of the imagination, the placebo effect and the comfort that one may get from an illusion. Jorge had always been a sensible, intelligent family man who engaged, out of desperation as do many in his situation, in a fantasy.

What to do with that *witch doctor* and so many others like him? The ethical answer is an easy one; the legal one is not, which explains why there are so many individuals still selling chimeras and useless, harmful products. Ethically, they are clearly immoral; legally, they are difficult to prosecute because they hide under the protection of free speech.

Chelating agents, ionized water, bicarbonate and a myriad of unproven nutrients have been proposed by con artists and also by professionals gone amiss, to cure all types of ailments. In this last category, the most famous of them is Linus Pauling, who won the Nobel Prize in Chemistry in 1954 and later the Nobel Prize for peace. In 1970 he started advocating the use of mega doses of vitamins, especially Vitamin C, to combat all sorts of infirmities, from the common cold to cancer. Out of respect to his stature the Mayo Clinic conducted several studies to either corroborate or correct Pauling's claims. It was not surprising that all of his assertions proved wrong but more astonishing is the fact that he still has his followers, who every day consume inordinate amounts of vitamin C. Linus Pauling had an honest conviction and no intention to defraud the public, but something impaired his intellect and judgment.

There are some complementary means that are helpful in combating sickness, like certain foods which, through their intrinsic properties, prevent inflammation, oxidation, mutations and other changes, as we will discuss later. Nutrition is an exciting field that contributes to the understanding and prevention of disease, but unscrupulous individuals take ownership of certain ideas, twist them and use them for financial gain.

Let's take, for example, pomegranate, which has been extensively used on the Indian subcontinent as a panacea for all kinds of ailments for hundreds of years and now is becoming very popular in the US thanks to a heavy promotion and ongoing experimental and clinical studies. It has been advertised as a nutritional supplement useful in bleeding control; improving skin texture and muscle tone; improving heart function; curing hemorrhoids; preventing eye cataracts, hypertension and dental plaque; and having anticancer properties. Although this fruit and its derivatives are an excellent source of vitamins, antioxidants, potassium, polyphenols and phytochemicals, among other substances, none of the claims have been validated by sound scientific data. The FDA has warned different companies that the beneficial claims are still premature. In the meantime, pomegranate may be considered as well as consuming other fruits and vegetables rich in antioxidant activity.

One of my patients, the owner of a popular herbal store in Pasadena, CA, refused diagnostic tests in spite of severe symptoms; she was convinced that she could not be harboring a disease since she had been taking medicinal plants for most of her life; a year later, when she agreed to have an examination, she was found to be affected with late stage intestinal cancer.

Myths, fictions and deceptions are fed by the need we have to believe that something out there may magically make an infirmity go away, or make us fit, strong and healthy. While these aspirations stay in an abstract sphere they are innocuous, but brought to the physical world they can harm or kill us.

In other fields, safety concerns don't allow external forces to interfere. Aviation is an area guided by incontrovertible science and proven technological experimentation. Nothing leaves the ground unless facts have been tested and deemed safe. No interference by outsiders is allowed in building and running a plane. The administration, the supervision and the handling of the aviation industry is in the hands of experts and as a result flying is one of the safest pursuits. Medicine, on the other hand, although considered a strict discipline run by proficient professionals, is an open playing field hindered by thousands of non-professionals who engage without any authority in the delivery of care. This may come as a surprise but in the next pages you will learn who they are and what they do with total impunity. To make things worse, the provision of care, being a multidisciplinary undertaking, is also tainted by the same ones that are supposed to protect patients, being doctors, pharmaceutical companies and others.

We live under the illusion that when it comes to what we eat, what we breathe, or the medications we take, everything is fine, but it is not. If this seems like an exaggeration, just remember that in spite of all the advances in technology we are contracting infirmities of all kinds, more than ever before.

2

Myths in general are harmless and may even give flavor to life, by providing joy, comfort and delight.

My mother would never allow my siblings or me to go swimming unless one full hour passed after we had eaten. Otherwise, she told us, we would get stomach cramps and severe diarrhea. When I asked if that was a myth, she replied no, it was common knowledge and an accepted truth, period.

Watermelon and wine did not mix because the pulp of the fruit would trap alcohol for several hours and make our stomach bloated. That was my mother again.

From age 6 to 12 the kids in my family would be sent to summer camp; every Wednesday at bedtime we were given castor oil by Madame Kemp, the director of the retreat, to "clean our digestive system and get rid of toxins, poisons and harmful bacteria." Thursday mornings the facility was embedded in a rhapsody of smells that dissipated at noon. Laxatives as gut cleaners are a persistent myth.

Fanny, my aunt, cooked cabbage soup at least three times a week, because it cleaned the kidneys. Coming from her, a revered figure in our family, we took it as a sacrosanct credence.

Dionysus was the god of wine and resurrection in Greek Mythology, worshipped by many for centuries; today he remains only as a symbol of pleasurable libations and a myth long gone.

Others myths appear to be here to stay:

One that started in the 1800s and persists today is the belief that 13 is an unlucky number. If this belief is taken to extremes it is said that the sufferer is affected with a syndrome called (are you ready?) triskaidekaphobia.

Here are other myths that are part of the western culture, some of them unpretentious and harmless, others damaging:

We should fast on a periodic basis.

Whether nibbling is a better way to stay slim and healthy is still open to debate. Cher, the iconic singer, actress and director, will seldom eat a full meal; she prefers taking small bites 6 to 8 times a day as a way to stay trim. At age 65 she has the body and appearance of a much younger person; she probably is consuming the right amount of calories and good quality food, which explains the shape she is in and her energy. Independent of the frequency of her food intake, she has managed to stay fit and healthy.

Others are convinced that fasting on a regular basis detoxifies the body of impurities and is the way to stay well and strong. In this context the concept of detoxification is not well understood and a confusing one. Strictly speaking, to detoxify is to remove or decrease toxins from the body but unless we are sick we don't carry toxins or poisons in our body. Lead causes a condition called plumbism; iron overload, hemochromatosis; and mercury intoxication, neurological damage. In excess these substances are toxic and removing them from the body is clearly an accepted and proven mode of detoxification. Fasting is not a detoxifying method.

In 2005 Mark Mattson from the Laboratory of Neurosciences at Johns Hopkins ran a study on the effect of size and frequency of meals in relationship to health and longevity in rats. This experimental study was trying to assess if excessive energy intake is associated with cardiovascular disease, diabetes and cancer. He found that caloric restriction and reduced meal frequency and intermittent fasting can increase life span in rodents by reducing oxidative damage and by increasing stress resistance. Intermittent fasting resulted in increased production of a brain-derived neurotrophic factor that increased the resistance to neurological dysfunction and halted degenerative changes in animals. The process of fasting brought beneficial effects in these animals. For better understanding: the oxidative damage in the brain mentioned above would be like the corrosion of any material that is exposed to the air for long periods of time. Whether Mattson's experiments can be extrapolated to humans remains to be shown, but it is an interesting and revolutionary concept that may call upon us to drastically change our eating habits, something that may not ever happen because changing eating habits is a very difficult proposal and would require a profound cultural transformation.

Although there is no conclusive data about the benefits of fasting or nibbling or eating at different intervals, doing so would do no harm providing that the edibles contain the proper ingredients to meet the daily nutritional requirements and calorie intake matches calorie expenditure.

3

Some nutrients have a protective influence on longevity, memory and/or emotions and wine is to be cherished.

Fish, red wine, broccoli, olive oil, green tea and vegetables, among others, have a reputation for making people healthier and prolonging life. Some of them have enjoyed lasting respect, while others are long forgotten. Fish, for example, have maintained a reputation as one of the healthiest foods available. Other studies have been done on the dietary habits and lifestyles of centenarians in different societies, with the idea to replicate their habits to reap the same benefits.

Some nutrients are believed to improve cognition. Fernando Gomez-Pinilla, a UCLA professor of neurosurgery, believes that food is often more effective than supplements when it comes to brain health. He investigated the effect of different substances on cognition. His theory is that diet manipulation may increase the resistance of neurons to external insult and promote mental fitness. Others claim that certain amino acids may help the production of neurotransmitters linked to prevent depression.

Food may become a magic potion that can preserve brain function intact or in the worst of cases delay the process of brain aging, conserving our memory, learning skills and emotional stability. The subtle hope behind food manipulation is preventing Alzheimer's and other brain degenerative disease. To die at old age with an intact mentation is a most cherished aspiration.

Joel C. Robertson, the author of *Natural Prozac*, believes that Vitamins B6 and B12 play an important role in converting amino acids into neurotransmitters like serotonin and norepinephrine and preventing depression. He may be right, but this does not mean that if people are depressed they should ingest B6 and B12 supplements, since we get more than our daily requirement of these vitamins by eating, beef, turkey, fruits, vegetables, eggs, chicken and shellfish.

The attributes of the following edibles, once mythical, are a matter of fact but one should not read more into what they tell:

Fish: Different fishes have different properties but almost all are an excellent source of proteins. Saltwater fish, mainly salmon, herring trout, anchovy, sardines, white fish and sablefish, are rich in Omega-3 fatty acids, which are known to decrease the incidence of cardiovascular disease.

Japanese eat fish in large amounts and have long lifespan. Women in Japan live an average of 85 years and men 78, some of the highest in the world. Whether it is fish or other products like tofu, soy, and wheat and buckwheat flour, green tea and/or eating smaller portions (which is part of their eating habits) are the main factor to their longevity is an open question. Dr. Dean Ornish and other serious scientists are big proponents of eating fish, although selectively. If fish is not available, it is possible to take three grams a day of supplemental Omega 3, which is usually well tolerated and has few side effects.

Red Wine: "It is an absolute myth that red wine is good for you," says Valerie Beral from Oxford University and the author of the *Million Women Study*. According to Dr. Beral only one drink a week increases the incidence of cancers of the breast, pharynx and liver in women. But Dr. Roger Corder from William Harvey Research Institute in England and author of the *Red Wine Diet* strongly disagrees. He says that certain red wines containing a group of flavonoid polyphenols, containing procyanadins are cardio protective. He claims that is not resveratrol, another antioxidant present in wine that provides those benefits, since it has too minimal a presence to be relevant. Dr. Corder warns to be selective in choosing wine, since there are not that many that contain procyanadins in sufficient amounts. The good ones are from France and Sardinia and other regions. Males from Sardinia live longer than any other population group in the world; the fact that they drink red wine routinely may or may not account for their prolonged existence. Sardinians also eat a lot of goat cheese, so is cheese what accounts for their long survival? Or is it the Y-chromosome's haplogroup, which is carried by almost half of the population?

It is tempting to accept wine as a source of longevity and drink one or two glasses of wine every day and live happily and longer ever after. But keep in mind that two respectable scientists, from two respectable institutions, have different opinions about the topic. My recommendation is to drink red wine rich in procyanadins once a day, while women with a personal or family history or genetic makeup for breast cancer, should avoid alcohol altogether until more science about the subject comes along. Also, note that chocolate, Red Delicious and Granny Smith apples and cranberry juice contain more procyanadins than wine.

Green tea: This ancient concoction is the latest craze and lots of people are jumping on board to exploit its potential economic rewards. Booths in malls, vendors in supermarkets, and commercials all over the media are some of the means to entice us to consume green tea, which is now becoming purportedly the potion of eternal youth. The supporters of green tea believe that drinking four cups a day decreases the risk of cardiovascular disease, reduces blood pressure, improves cognition, and slows down the progression of Parkinson's, Alzheimer's and Multiple Sclerosis. They claim that it is an excellent adjuvant for weight loss and that it decreases cholesterol by slowing the flow of pancreatic juice or down-regulating post-prandial glucose. Green tea contains antioxidants and polyphenols, which in animal experimentation have shown to confer protection to the heart and the brain. These claims are irresistibly appealing and encouraging, albeit unproven. Currently there are multiple studies assessing the protective properties of green tea on the above-mentioned areas and also on diabetes and breast, ovarian and prostate cancer

A review article published in *Liver International and* comprised of a Medline search, Embase database and Chinese scientific journals came to the conclusion that some of the assertions may be valid. In the June 7, 2009 online edition of GUT, an actuarial analysis showed that women who drink five cups of green tea a day have decreased incidence of gastric cancer but there were some confounders in the reviewed studies, such as dosage and design that do not allow concluding definitively that green tea is a miracle brew.

Since green tea is not expensive and used by millions with no apparent side effects, there is no contraindication to its consumption.

Broccoli: This is an excellent vegetable containing fiber and vitamins with probably potent anti-cancer properties. Victoria Kirsch and collaborators in a recent article published in *The Journal of the National Cancer Institute* suggested that it reduces the incidence of aggressive cancer of the prostate. Dr. Paul Evans showed that broccoli and related vegetables may have a protective effect on the heart by the presence of sulphoraphane, a naturally occurring biochemical found in relative abundance in fresh broccoli. An article published in *Cancer Prevention Research* claims that broccoli protects against cancer of the stomach.

Olive oil: Olive oil is the god of all oils. To some it is magical. Its fascination comes from being cardio protective and enhancing longevity. It contains monounsaturated fat, mainly oleic acid, which was shown to decrease the level of cholesterol in the blood; it has anti-inflammatory properties; and it decreases blood pressure. It also contains polyphenol, a powerful antioxidant, which has been shown to increase arterial elasticity. There are other unsubstantiated claims that it may prevent cancer and other degenerative conditions and that it may increase insulin sensitivity, thus helping to reduce diabetes. It is rich in Vitamin E, which also has antioxidant properties. In contrast with animal oils, it does not contain trans-fats (which increase cholesterol and triglycerides). It is rich in Omega-3 fatty acids, which protect against heart attacks and strokes.

It has antiplatelet activity, like aspirin, and anti-inflammatory properties like ibuprofen. Olive oil comes in different shapes and forms: extra-virgin, virgin, pure and refined. In the US it is classified as Grade A to Grade D. Extra-virgin is best, as it is Grade A. The taste and the aroma depend on the soil where the olive trees grow, the method of harvesting and the process of elaboration, like being cold pressed within hours of harvesting. The freshness of the olive oil is important because after being stored for more than one year it loses its flavor and the beneficial qualities.

Two tablespoonfuls a day is the minimum recommended amount.

Greeks, Italians, Spaniards and people from the Middle East are the largest consumers of olive oil. They use it generously in almost everything they eat. One may indulge with no guilt when consuming olive oil, although it contains 120 calories in each tablespoonful.

Canola Oil has long been neglected; it is rich in Omega-6 and has been proven to decrease the risk of coronary artery disease. This oil comes from cross-breeding several types of rape plants from the mustard family, along with turnips, watercress, radish, horseradish and cabbage.

Mediterranean diet effectively prolongs life span:

The word Mediterranean has a nice connotation attached to it. It reminds one of a place with beautiful coastlines, pleasant weather, evergreen trees, blue waters, sea turtles and not least a cuisine that takes advantage of the richness of their soil and surrounding waters, endowing its inhabitants with foods that are consistently healthful and tasteful time after time, an enviable combination.

There is a longstanding belief that a Mediterranean diet, which consists of high intake of vegetables, legumes, fruits, and cereals; high intake of unsaturated fatty acids, mostly in the form of olive oil; low intake of saturated fatty acids; moderately high intake of fish; low to moderate intake of dairy products, mostly as cheese or yogurt; low intake of meat or poultry and a regular but moderate amount of red wine, protects against coronary artery disease, hypertension, diabetes, obesity and cancer and prolongs lifespan.

One study led by N. Scarmeas from Columbia University Medical Center showed that adherence to a Mediterranean diet, coupled with high level of physical activity, was independently associated with a lower incidence of Alzheimer's disease. This was corroborated by another similar study in Bordeaux, France, by C. Feart. Both articles were published in *The Journal of the American Medical Association.*

For the last 20 years serious scientific research conducted to elicit the goodness of the Mediterranean diet has shown that has a significant protective health effect.

Chicken Soup cures the common flu:

Who can doubt that chicken soup can help in fighting a cold? For centuries it has also been claimed to combat the flu. Chicken soup has been a matter of research by scientists, material for writers and the stuff of philosophers. Some physicians have shown that it clears the passage of mucus from the nose, others that activates white cells to fight inflammation and others that it has potent anti-infection properties. A simple explanation of its merits is the idea that it provides hydration and salt, which is needed when a person becomes sick and is unable to eat or drink normally.

Others claim that it cures asthma, hypertension, thyroiditis and other ailments. These are anecdotal stories that have roots in this ancient tradition advocated by Maimonides, the 12ᵗʰ century physician and philosopher who advocated consuming fowl in different forms, including soup, to cure all kinds of ailments, including leprosy, asthma and infections. Truth or fiction, it has earned a deserved place among our cultural traditions. But to qualify as a panacea it has to be prepared by your mother.

4

These myths and so many others are awaiting their final sanction. Will red wine became the elixir of health, broccoli the most venerated vegetable on earth, green tea the magic potion and Mediterranean food a universal diet? We may not have yet an absolute answer, but we can assert that using olive oil, eating broiled fish, a potpourri of fruits and vegetables or a luscious Mediterranean dish should be encouraged. To wait for scientific studies, which will be welcome, makes no sense because the time for wellness is now. It should not be rigorous scientific data or on the other hand foolish food designs that should dictate what we eat. It should not be a guilty conscience that shapes our eating habits but rather a determined sense of purpose of being mindful that eating the right stuff is a sound investment in health. The road to good health always comes down to eating well, exercising and being emotionally stable, simple paradigms that we will be repeating again and again in this book. They are the light that illuminates our spiritual journey to be and stay healthy.

5

Lies are like flies: they are everywhere, annoying and disturbing. When it comes to medicine lies are dreadful. There is a multitude of dishonest persons trying to make money in the health arena, from innocent people.

One purpose of this book is to provide the reader with tools to achieve optimal health and alert them to the scammers who are everywhere. It would be impossible to list all the tricks and falsehoods that are out there; therefore, I will list only some that are unfortunately accepted and practiced by many. I have already mentioned some machinations from the food industry; later, I will be discussing acts of dishonesty by professionals and pharmaceutical companies.

I am not asserting that there is a conspiracy of sorts by some to maim us or subvert an established order, yet in the quest to make money they do disregard safety and good practice.

Many individuals, institutions and corporations unethically, albeit legally, are maiming our wellbeing. Here are some of those scams:

The colon is full of toxins that should be removed.

About 10 years ago I saw a 42 year old patient in my office with a history of moderate abdominal pain and a definitive change in bowel habits for more than a year. She was first seen by a "health advisor," a self-proclaimed individual who had been dispensing herbs and other services in Venice, California, who recommended colon cleansing treatments every two weeks. After one year her symptoms got worse, so she decided to seek a formal gastroenterological consultation. I performed several tests that showed that she had a colon cancer which had already metastasized to the liver and other structures; she received palliative treatment and died few months later. This is not an infrequent case, where uncalled-for practices delay diagnosis at an early stage of the disease. If she had been seen earlier perhaps she should be alive today.

Colon cleansing, or colon therapy, as it is also called, is one of the most egregious and flagrant violations to the human body. The idea of removing toxins from the intestine has no scientific foundation. This practice is advertised as a cure for arthritis, sinus problems, fatigue, depression, obesity, constipation, belly size reduction, foul breath, backaches, mood swings and to improve the immune system. Not one of these claims has a scientific basis or pragmatic validity. In spite of being disregarded by the medical community as scams, its practice is flourishing.

Colon cleansing is performed by water enemas containing different products like coffee, vitamins, laxatives like cascara, herbs and other substances, or   by ingesting cleansing products, none of which have proven efficacy. These practices are endorsed by celebrities, the same ones who are desperately seeking the fountain of youth in the form of pills, creams, body manipulation and plastic surgery. They are heavily promoted by fashion publishers because writing about these fat busters, magical anti-wrinkle creams, pills to provide a youthful appearance, detoxification programs and other nonsense promises, sells magazines.

The American Cancer Society states, "Available scientific evidence does not support claims that colon therapy is effective in treating cancer or any other disease. Colon therapy can be dangerous and can cause infection or death."

In 1985, The California Department of Health Services listed the following known hazards of colon therapy: infection and death from contaminated equipment; death from electrolyte depletion and puncture of the intestine wall, leading to life-threatening sepsis or death. They neglected to mention the harm of delaying a diagnosis, as we have seen in my young patient. So, why are we then still allowing this dreadful practice? It is a puzzling question.

The function of the colon is to remove water from our body and absorb and secrete electrolytes as a way to keep a normal balance of these vital constituents. It is a reservoir of the residuals arriving from the small intestine, which are finally eliminated as feces. Stool elimination is carried out at different intervals, depending on amount and quality of ingested food. The indigestible material such as fiber provides the bulk of the stool, which also contains, water, salts, bacteria and other materials. Trillions of bacteria are lodged in the colon, and they live in the perfect balance needed to maintain proper function. Tampering its operation is a risky intrusion into bodily function. Persons with cardiac problems may develop water intoxication from enemas; others develop water and electrolyte disturbance from the frequent use of laxatives. Other complications include rectal or intestinal perforation. Not infrequently, dependency develops and this leads to constipation. Laxatives mixed with herbs may interfere with absorption of needed nutrients. Three cases of death have been reported in the US after the use of colon hydrotherapy. The idea to implement this nonsense practice started centuries ago as a means of cleaning our 'sewage system'. Laxatives and enemas were routinely recommended to prevent accumulation of waste, but waste in the colon is a normal state of affairs. This practice is popular because it creates the illusion of eliminating poisons from our body.

6

Some advocates of alternative or complementary medicine use illusions and deceptions to treat a variety of chronic diseases or unresolved medical issues. They resort to herbs, dietary supplements, vitamins, minerals and diet manipulation, promising a cure that they never deliver.

In a way we are their accomplices, because in our quest for good health we do silly things and surrender to our fantasies. For many who have been diagnosed with an intractable condition, it is difficult to resist the promise that there may be something else, not proven yet, that may reverse or halt a condition. It is hard to take away hope when the reality is hopeless.

There are complementary treatments proven to help patients who suffer with cancer or other chronic medical conditions, like meditation to reduce stress, marijuana to relieve nausea or vomiting from chemotherapy, relaxation techniques, massage therapy, or mental exercises to enhance the medical effectiveness of conventional drugs and the body immune response, but palliation and temporary comfort should not be confused with cure.

Evidence in medicine does not come quickly; it is only after large clinical trials that we can assert that a procedure or pharmacological agent works well enough to be adopted by the entire medical community.

Medical science should be held in high regard, but with the understanding that although it has contributed enormously in providing cures to otherwise fatal conditions, alleviating all kind of ailments, prolonging life and making life better, this discipline does not have the last word in the subject of health, either. **This is why some feel entitled to fill that void.**

The shortcomings of conventional medicine should be emphasized; we are still making one million medical errors and as a consequence 90,000 people die every year; we are still relying more on writing a prescription than putting emphasis in lifestyle modification; we are not giving prevention proper consideration; we are subjecting patients to unnecessary tests, either for fear of malpractice litigation or because that is where the money is. Medications are imperfect and many of them are being recalled after having produced irreversible damage or death. Some pharmaceutical companies use their marketing skills to entice people to consume medications as if they were candy.

And worse, we are medicalizing natural processes. If our skin becomes wrinkled as we age, they promise a cure for something that cannot and does not need a cure. If we don't sleep at night because we have a worry, a sleeping pill is prescribed instead of trying to understand where the anxiety is coming from and how to deal with it on an emotional level. If you are a woman and your libido is down because of an annoying, difficult relationship you may be suffering from a new, recently invented syndrome, 'female sexual desire disorder,' for which testosterone is indicated. Testosterone, a medication not exempt from serious side effects, is now a billion dollar business for treatment of a condition that does not exist.

7

A succinct list of deceptions:

In the early years of cell phones, Martin Cooper, who developed the first portable phone, testified before a Michigan commission that driving while talking on the phone carried significant physical risk. This was when cell phones were not that popular. His contention proved to be correct. In spite of this, the cell companies dismissed the problem, claiming that those assertions were unfounded; only after collected data from a Harvard study showed that cell phones or texting causes 570,000 accidents and 2,600 fatalities every year did they come around and accept that this practice is dangerous and renounce their previous position. The prohibition to drive and talk on the phone is costing the cell companies millions of dollars, which explains their early efforts to conceal how hazardous it could be. Other big industries obscured their practices to protect their profits. GlaxoSmithKline failed to disclose that Paxil could cause suicidal thoughts in children and agreed to a 2.5 million dollar settlement, as revealed in an article published in the *New York Times* on May 31, 2005. Vioxx was removed from the market because it caused fatal heart attacks, and apparently the results of clinical trials showing this fact were known by the manufacturer. Dr. Marcia Angell, the former editor in chief of the *New England Journal of Medicine*, the author of the book *The Truth about the Drug Companies* and a reform health advocate wrote, "...Over the past two decades the pharmaceutical industry has moved very far from its original high purpose of discovering and producing useful new drugs. Now primarily a marketing machine to sell drugs of dubious benefits, this industry uses its wealth and power to co-opt every institution that might stand in its way, including the US Congress, the FDA, academic medical centers and the medical profession itself."

Dioxin use in animal feedings was found to be carcinogenic, in spite of which, according to Eric Pianin from *The Washington Post,* "....the chemical, beef and poultry industries are waging an intense campaign to delay further an Environmental Protection Agency study showing that consumption of animal fat and dairy products containing traces of dioxin can cause cancer in humans."

Corporations, at times, prefer to collect profits, hiding potential harm from their products, be it arsenic in drinking water or chemicals in their food offerings.

In previous chapters we mentioned that in order to increase preservation of food, and palatability the food industry uses preservatives, dyes, genetic manipulation, and chemicals to change color and texture and reengineering techniques. This results in a hybrid that resembles food but is really an artificial compound generically known as processed food.

A chicken nugget is a dysmorphic piece of chopped chicken with all its components, the skin included, to which fillers, fat and breading is added and cooked in hydrogenated oil. The consumer believes that since it is 'chicken' it is healthy. As a result they (most of whom are kids below the age of 6) get 250 calories in one serving, half of them coming from fat.

There are plenty of other foodstuffs that are not what they appear to be. Thousands of processed foods present on the shelves of the supermarket are phony concoctions. In general they contain one ingredient that gives the name to the meal, for example steak, but looking carefully at the components, it is clear the mixture is far from being a steak but rather is a new construct, an industrially created food.

Added artificial flavor is also a deception; French fries may taste very good due more to added chemicals and unnatural ingredients than to the quality of the potato; it is not the Idaho soil that gives them flavor but rather a chemical factory in New Jersey. Strawberry ice cream may not contain one miniscule part of the fruit, just artificial flavors, enough to create an illusion that tricks our senses. Not too long ago I saw a lemonade drink in a dispenser that carried a label that said "contains no lemonade"!

Meat is not infrequently recalled when it is contaminated with E. coli 0157:H7, a virulent bacterium that produces severe disease—the uremic hemolytic syndrome—which has a mortality rate of around 10 percent. Each year about 76 million people get sick from food infestation with bacteria, viruses or parasites present in raw meat during slaughter, handling or preparation before it arrives to your kitchen. Foodborne illnesses are not uncommon. The Produce Safety Project at Georgetown University reported in March of 2010 that this costs 152 billion dollars a year, including medical care, loss of productivity and wages, which gives an idea of the magnitude of the problem. At times food poisoning is due to casual infestation passed from food handlers at the end of the chain of the food supply, or from a supermarket, a restaurant or home preparation. In other instances it is due to poor practices in the food industry, such as lack of sanitary control, processing or inadequate testing. This calamity is only now being addressed by Congress, which is considering different bills to confront the problem of food safety.

In the book *Food Inc.,* we read, "We have secretive corporations that increasingly control not just the food supply but the very genetic makeup of the plants that sustain life on Earth" and they add "... the American food production system and its impact on our health, our economy and even our freedoms as a people is a theme with vast ramifications."

Our long-established eating routines are being replaced by new ones by the slow and pervasive actions of powerful food manufacturers. We may think that we are free to choose what we eat, but we may not be, because we are being manipulated by the food industry, which through their advertisements, marketing practices and artificially created trends, entice us to eat what in the long run will harm us. Choice and decision making are complex tasks. Jonah Lehrer, a Rhodes Scholar who worked in the lab of the Nobel Prize-winning neuroscientist Eric Kandel, wrote in his book *How We Decide* that dopamine, the neurotransmitter, is released when we eat and this is tied to predictable outcomes. If we eat what we like, the neurons fire dopamine and these results in a positive emotion; on the contrary, if one does not get an anticipated reward, dopamine release shuts off and we feel unhappy. It is this link of prediction tied to our emotions that dictates how we behave in general. When we eat we start a process of decision making based on a cycle of prediction and reward. Eating something very appetizing creates a cycle difficult to break. The food industry knows this very well, and that is why they offer palatable, tasty, inexpensive edibles aimed at our emotions; in this way previous experience, mistakes, predictions and expectations dictate our behavior. If the food industry gets it right, we get hooked. No longer has our reason to eat what is right prevailed, but rather the memory of what in the past gave us so much pleasure. This has created a gestalt where the predominant foodstuffs are full of fat, sugar and salt, a mixture of unhealthy proportions but difficult to resist.

There is a group of physicians, educators, nutritionists and investigative journalists who are urging people to return to basic, natural, sound eating habits. Peter Pringle, Arthur Rodriguez, Michael Pollan and others are trying to bring clarity to the eating quandary. They point to the fact that sound farming practices are coming to an end, that animals are being fed in cages and are not pasturing in the fields and that corn has become the main ingredient in their feedings, replacing healthier nourishment.

Fortunately, organic, whole, and natural foods are being reintroduced and new habits, where processed foods have no place, are encouraged. State and federal agencies are embarking on campaigns promoting healthy eating habits not different from the fight against drugs and tobacco.

Deception can be found in the fast food eateries, where they display enticing products in such a way that they end up betraying our common sense. Their commercials create the illusion that they offer the best expressions of culinary art.

Burger King, complying with federal and local regulations, offers nutritional information about their products in a brochure that should prompt a conscious consumer to question the safety of certain products.

One example among the 53 foodstuffs they sell is their **specialty bun.** According to an information sheet, the buns contain the following ingredients:

...enriched unbleached wheat flour (wheat flour, malted barley flour or alpha amylase from Aspergillus Orizae, niacin, iron, thiamine mononitrate (vitamin B1) Riboflavin (vitamin B12, folic acid, ascorbic acid, water, high fructose-corn syrup or liquid sucrose, yeast, vegetable oil Canola and/or soy) or soybean and/or cottonseed oil. May contain less than 2 % or less of the following: salt, vital wheat gluten, soy flour, cornstarch, yeast nutrient (may contain one or more of the following: ammonium sulfate, monocalcium phosphate, calcium sulfate, calcium carbonate, Dicalcium sulfate) dough conditioners (may contain one or more of the following: wheat starch, microcrystalline cellulose, sorbitol, sodium stearoyl lactylate, ascorbic acid, azodicarbonamide, mono and diglycerides, calcium peroxide, calcium stearoyl-2 lacylate,datem),enzymes, preservatives(calcium propionate and/or sorbic acid, vinegar, sesame seeds, cellulose gel, leavening (sodium acid pyrophosphate, sodium bicarbonate, diammonium phosphate.) Does not contain animal products.

How different from the bread that my grandparents cooked in their bakery using only flour, water, salt, and yeast, which tasted so much better than these fluffy fabrications!

If these popular food joints with thousands and thousands of stores were to manufacture bread in their local premises they would not need to use chemicals and preservatives, but the price of the bun would be higher, cutting into their profits. The same goes for each single product they sell. They have mastered the technique of mass production, which brought with it the creation of **food-like stuff,** which looks and tastes good (because of fat, salt and sugar) but contains harmful substances. For the industry the numbers are clear, saving 10 cents in one burger and selling 10 million of them translates into a profit of 1,000,000 dollars. Since people consume millions of burgers a day, you do the math.

The deception comes from the fantasy that if one discloses the ingredients there is nothing to fear, like the fine print on a document that nobody reads. Few people read posted notices about food composition, or its warnings.

There are no good reasons to patronize fast food joints and yet we do because their enticements are difficult to resist. McDonald's, Burger King, Wendy's and other food joints are part of our culture and recognized all over the world as staples of American cuisine. The stores are colorful; the food is cheap and tasty. We use them as a system of reward and punishment. If kids get good grades, finish their homework on time or keep their room clean they are rewarded with a trip to McDonald's, Cheesy Cheek, Burger King or others. There they get meals, collectibles, and discounted passes to Disneyland, baseball cards and toys. This creates a cycle of anticipation and rewards, a steady one, assuring an involuntary association: eat-be happy-eat again and again... Some fast food places have a playground, a way to lure customers to come, consume and play. Attendance at these joints is always very good, even in times of economic crisis, when penny pinching is a must. Their businesses have no flaws.

Fortunately, there are some relentless health watchers that are demanding fast food chains change their ways and become aware of the health implications of what they serve. For example, Dr. Dean Ornish was hired as a consultant for McDonald's and has advised them to stop the use of saturated oils.

Children's obesity is reaching epidemic proportions, and it is imperative to take a strong stand and demand that foods served in public places are not hypercaloric or of little nutritional value. The three larger soft drink corporations have now removed high calorie drinks from the vending machines in schools and replaced them with others without carbohydrates.

Fast food eateries are ingrained in our civilization and will not go away. They are part of our way of life. It shouldn't be that difficult to become creative and transform them into places where kids could enjoy good food and have fun. Developing an ethos of respect for people's health will benefit their business and our wellbeing. One case in point: Coke is now offering small cans of their beverages, a commendable action, since less volume translates into fewer calories, and yet some fast food joints are offering 24 oz. cups of soft drinks, providing a whopping 420 calories.

If you think that I and those who are warning about the perils and hazards of food are exaggerating their claims, think again. Let's read further in Burger King's brochure:

Warning – Chemicals known to the state of California to cause cancer or birth defects or other reproductive harm may be present in foods or beverages sold or serve here. Cooked potatoes that have been browned, such as French Fries, hash browns and Cheesy Tots potatoes contain acrylamide, a chemical known to the state of California to cause cancer.

This chemical is not added to our foods but is created when certain foods are browned. Other foods sold here, such as hamburger buns, biscuits, croissants and coffee, also contain acrylamide, but generally in lower concentration than fried potatoes. Your personal cancer risk is affected by a wide variety of factors. The FDA has not advised people to stop eating baked or fried potatoes. For more information see **www.fda.gov**.

Some foods served here may contain other chemicals formed as a byproduct of cooking that are known to cause cancer or birth defects or other reproductive harm. These chemicals include polycyclic aromatic hydrocarbons and Phip (2-amino-1-metyl-6-phenylimidazol (4, 5, b) pyridine (in grilled chicken).

Burger King is not concealing anything and is complying with governmental regulations in disclosing the content of their food. And here is where the deception comes. The fact that fast food joints are open for business is a tacit illusion of the safety of their products. A recent study from New York University and Yale performed at McDonald's, Burger King, Kentucky Fried Chicken and Wendy's showed that calorie postings in restaurants do not change people's habits, consistent with the perception that people buy what is best for their money, independent of health considerations.

This brings us to the subject of individual responsibility, a subject that is not as simple as it looks because of the interplay of multiple variants, which are dependent on socioeconomic status, education, cultural background, sex, age, previous experience, societal norms, religious convictions, philosophical belief, mental status, opportunity and the freedom to choose.

We are easy to condemn those who eat the wrong stuff all the time and who consequently develop a sickness, but some have limited economic means and can only get satiated by consuming empty calories with little nutritional value because of its low price.

It is the society as a whole and the food industry in particular who should be accountable for bad practices.

This is reminiscent of the early stages of tobacco consumption, when smoking was glamorous and a sign of masculinity. There was no real understanding of the harm of nicotine until the early 40s. After that time the consumers, the government, health organizations, health providers and the rest of us took notice that smoking causes cancer of the lungs and bladder; cardiovascular and cerebrovascular disease; and emphysema and slowly started to take action to decrease the consumption of cigarettes, but not without a fight from the manufacturers.

At the beginning they hid data that showed the harmful effects of smoking, denied adding extra nicotine to enhance addiction, engaged in shameful marketing practices and refused to acknowledge that tobacco caused cancer, which parallels what the food industry is doing today

Here is another example of a common practice that is more dangerous than we suspected. Atrazine is a weed killer that is used on corn fields and is contaminating our drinking water. This herbicide appears to be responsible for birth defects, low birth weights and reproductive problems and perhaps cancer at concentrations previously approved by the Environmental Protection Agency. In spite of this and against the advice of environmentalists, some in the agriculture industry are still utilizing it on their fields, passing it into fruit and vegetables and then to us.

The disclosure practices are treacherous because a disclaimer is not enough to prevent people from using a hazardous substance. Cigarette packaging clearly has a warning about its product, as food manufacturers do. The ethical connotations are clear. It is morally wrong to sell something that may be damaging to individuals when 90 percent of the evidence shows that it is.

We go to fast food joints and we take our children along without understanding the harm associated with eating the wrong stuff, because the offenders don't make us sick right away; they kill very slowly, by making us fat, hypertensive, diabetic or cancer-prone.

8

Most popular diet books, diet pills and related paraphernalia are useless and expensive.

Other merchants of hope are those who, with or without any qualifications, take advantage of the niche that they see in the market for a miracle diet, a magic pill to curtail our appetite or whatever gimmick may arise from their imagination to convince the world that losing weight is at hand for the millions of overweight persons who are desperately seeking to become slim and slender. Since none of these books have been able to accomplish much, new ones appear every day in the shelves of bookstores.

There are two types of diet books: ones written by honest professionals and others by swindlers and charlatans.

A sensible, rational book offers sound, scientific and proven advice. An earnest diet books offers a well balanced, low calorie, easy to prepare, palatable and economical diet plan. The lists of foods include the permitted and the prohibited in terms of their nutritional value and their content; the statements are substantiated by verifiable facts, confirmed to be effective, and provide irrefutable health benefits

The differences among them are the recipes, composition and the way of cooking, but in the end all have a common denominator: **reducing calories while maintaining a proper nutritional balance.**

Since it is known that more than 80 percent of people fail in achieving their dietary goals, many serious and casual writers have been looking for twists to offer a miraculous diet that would require little personal effort. Low calorie diets are restrictive by definition and thus difficult to adhere to. In order to resolve this problem Dr. Robert Atkins created a low-carbohydrate diet which was permissive in other ways. Instead of focusing on calories it focused on content. It consisted of allowing liberal amounts of proteins and fat but no sugars. His book, *Dr. Atkins' Diet Revolution*, published in 1972 became a best seller. Millions of people bought the book and millions were able to shed a significant amount of pounds, albeit for a short period of time. His theory was that refined sugars, flour and high-fructose corn syrup were responsible for triggering obesity. He advocated eating proteins with minimal restriction. In doing this, he claimed, the body would burn stored body fat instead of sugars. His hypotheses were correct but with some caveats that proved to be harmful. A seminal study, published in the *New England Journal of Medicine (NEJM),* showed in 2003 that the Atkins Diet effectively decreased weight compared to a control group but only for the first three months, after which time patients started to gain weight again. In 2009 a group of investigators led by Dr. F.M. Sacks from Harvard School of Public Health performed a very important study, also published in the *NEJM.* They randomly assigned 811 overweight adults to one of four diets. The foods were similar in all groups but the concentration of fat, protein and carbohydrates varied from group to group. Patients were followed for two years. Eighty percent completed the study, an unusual accomplishment. All of them, in addition, attended instructional sessions. The primary goal was to evaluate the change in body weight comparing: low fat versus high fat and average protein intake and high protein and high and low carbohydrate content. At six months participants assigned to each diet had lost an average of 6 kg (13.2 lbs), and all began to regain weight after 12 months. By two years the average weight loss was 4 kg (8.8 lbs) but only 14 to 15% of the participants had a reduction of at least 10% of their initial body weight.

The bottom line was that **reduced-calorie diets** resulted in clinically meaningful weight loss, regardless of which macronutrients were provided. Fourteen to fifteen percent of those who were able to keep their weight down were quite an accomplishment. These subjects had the incentive of being part of a controlled experiment, were receiving counseling sessions, and their enrollment in the study probably meant that they started with a high motivation, which amounts to an artificial situation, difficult to duplicate in real life.

Severe restriction of carbohydrates appeared wrong to many. Dr. Robert Eckel of the American Heart Association stated unequivocally that **the Atkins diet puts people at risk of heart disease**.

Some diet books are written by dishonest or incompetent professionals, actors and actresses, opportunists and self-proclaimed gurus with two purposes: money and fame.

Catchy titles also help in selling books, some good and some bad, like *Flat Belly Diet*, *Paleolithic Diet*, *South Beach Diet*, *Beverly Hills Diet*, *Skinny Bitch* and similar ones have become best sellers, some lasting on the bookstore shelves longer than others. Famous household names get into the fray, becoming advocates for better health: Suzanne Somers (who remains slim) and Oprah Winfrey (who relapsed) are two from a long list of celebrities. Marie Osmond is now a spokesperson for Nutrisystem; if she stays fit she will retain that privilege, otherwise she will be dropped and be replaced by another celebrity, which is what happened to another actress, Kirstie Alley, who was dismissed by Jenny Craig after gaining back 75 pounds. Kirstie was replaced by Queen Latifah, who paradoxically also does commercials for Pizza Hut.

Mindful books that promote weight loss by recommending judicious low calorie, well balanced diets and encouraging lifestyle modification including burning excessive calories through controlled physical activities should be welcome and serve as a guide to carry people through the difficult intricacies of losing weight.

Others are silly, dangerous or both like the one that supports the ancient tradition of drinking urine to promote wellbeing or to be used as an anticancer agent. When these types of books become popular the medical community takes notice, raising valid criticism. The *Beverly Hills Diet* sold more than one million copies and was endorsed by famous actresses. Yet in 1981 an article by Dr. Gabe Mirkin of the University of Maryland, published in *The Journal of the American Medical Association,* criticized the diet for its potential harmful effects and wrote it was **"the latest and perhaps the worst entry in the diet-fad derby."**

Over the last decade or so the Internet has emerged as a powerful force that is shaping the way we eat and exercise, not to mention the influence it has on our lifestyle. Bloggers, professionals, non-professionals, good, bad, intelligent and injudicious people are somewhere in the Web Universe having their voice being heard and trying with good or bad intentions to make us change our way of life. Guidance and counsel are easy to come by, but without discernment they are harmful.

All these trappings will not go away; they are rooted in trying to find an easy way out to our desire to stay trim.

> Success in achieving your goals is never easy; it arises from inner energy and never from indolence.

9

Are there effective drugs in reducing weight?

Among the paraphernalia that people use to fight obesity are prescription drugs to curb appetite. Pharmaceutical companies spend inordinate amounts of money trying to develop a magic diet pill. Since people spend about 59 billion dollars a year to shed pounds, whoever finds the right alternative may take home a big chunk of that money.

There are two types of medications for weight loss. One is directed to decrease appetite and the other to decrease the absorption of fats, for example by inhibiting lipase, an enzyme that breaks down fat.

The available drugs in the US are:

Sibutramine, Orlistat, Phentermine, Diethylpropion, Fluoxetine, Sertraline, Bupropion, Topiramate and Zonisamide

Orlistat decreases the absorption of fat and by doing this produces diarrhea, flatulence, bloating and abdominal pain. Topiramate and Zonisamide work by an unknown mechanism but have at times significant side effects like paresthesias (sensorial changes like tingling or burning of the skin) and changes in taste for the former and somnolence, dizziness and nausea for the latter. All appetite suppressants have variable and at times significant side effects; they are unreliable and produce minimal or modest reduction in weight.

Effective appetite suppressants do not exist at this time; if one becomes available it will sell by the billions but will help only **temporarily,** since one cannot take them forever.

Fen-Phen was an anti-obesity medication, sold by the millions after being aggressively marketed, which became infamous for having killed or permanently damaged many people by destroying their lungs and their heart valves. The medication was withdrawn in 2004. Wyeth, the manufacturer, paid billions of dollars in damages. This underscores the need for prudence when taking these types of medications.

Contrave is a combination of Naitrexone and Bupropion, Iorcaserin and Qnexa a combination of Phentermine (Fen-Phen without the Fen, also known as flenfuramine). Clinical trials conducted for about a year showed better results than a placebo, with a range of weight loss between 5 and 10 percent. How are they going to work and how safe they would be in the long run, is anybody's guess.

Today, all pharmacological treatments for obesity are elusive, always temporary and in the long run probably ineffective.

The solution for the management of obesity lies in a rational diet, judicious physical exercise and stress management. Those are the foundations and, combined with other resources such as counseling, social support and professional interventions, are safe and effective.

10

Dietary and other supplements can help in promoting weight loss, fighting cancer and halting the progression of chronic ailments. Really?

Dietary supplements are many times deceiving, if not lethal. I have known this for many years, having seen a variety of products in Latin America, the United States and Europe containing chemicals that would induce weight loss but by artificial means and only temporarily; some of these products contain laxatives and diuretics, hence promoting weight loss by dehydration and depletion of electrolytes.

In the October 8, 2009 issue of the *NEJM*, Dr. Pieter Cohen published a paper, "American Roulette – Contaminated Dietary Supplements." The contamination was not only from bacteria, heavy metals and toxic plant material but from harmful substances like senna and cascara (laxatives) amphetamines (appetite suppressants) and others. Dr. Cohen raised the alarm because about 114 million people use dietary supplements. Since the supplements contain "natural" ingredients, they are considered safe and are free of scrutiny or regulation by governmental agencies. These products, marketed for patients with diabetes, high cholesterol, insomnia, sexual dysfunction, physical performance and weight loss, among many others, are either inefficient or pose a health hazard. The FDA found a stimulant (Sibutramine) in weight loss supplements at levels amounting to **three times the recommended dose**. Other substances present in some of the non-prescription herbs are rimonabant and fenproporex, which have been linked to suicide. Other ingredients in these compounds are benzodiazepines (used for panic disorders and anxiety), which have substantial side effects like cognitive impairment, aggression, violence and suicidal behavior. Others contain antidepressants, assuming that a mood lifting medication may decrease appetite, but because of its inefficiency and important side effects its use should be abandoned. To cover the presence of dangerous compounds the manufacturers use analogues, created by modifying the original chemical structure, making them difficult or impossible to detect. Regulation and active participation in curtailing the use of these masked substances by health agencies is lacking and as a consequence, injury and death occur in some patients.

The market for dietary supplements will not go away soon; on the contrary, it may increase because there is an eagerness among us to find simple, effective, quasi-magical substances to heal our ills. No matter what ailment we have, vendors are there; ready to sell magic cures to treat hypertension, prostate conditions, cancer, chronic degenerative diseases or others.

False claims and tainted herbal products muddy the waters of what is otherwise a legitimate field, which is the use of natural substances to prevent, ameliorate or cure certain conditions. Other natural substances, like turmeric (also known as curcumin) are safer and welcome in the armamentarium of healthy herbs. Turmeric is a shrub, related to ginger, which can be found in curry powders, cheeses and mustards. It is also called Indian saffron. In traditional Chinese and also Ayurvedic medicine, it has been used to aid digestion, improve liver function, ease arthritis, regulate menstrual period and fight cancer. Scientists have performed multiple experiments in rats and other animals inducing or transplanting malignant tumors showing unequivocally that turmeric either stops or reverses cancer progression. This inhibitory effect was shown in different cancers, including brain, colon, ovary, liver, stomach and leukemia. These results so far have been seen in **animal experimentation** but not in humans, an important distinction. Richard Beliveau in his laboratory at Sainte-Justine Children's Hospital in Montreal gave a cocktail of Brussels sprouts, broccoli, garlic, scallions, turmeric, black pepper, cranberry, grapefruit and green tea to immune-deprived mice and showed that they fare better in terms of motion, appetite and slow tumor growth when compared to a control group.

In India, the largest consumer of turmeric, the population has fewer incidences of colon, breast and lung cancers than those living in the West. Those features seem to suggest that this herb has significant therapeutic properties.

Now let's read what the National Institute of Health (NIH) says on their Web Page: "**...there is little evidence to support the use of turmeric for any health condition because few clinical trials have been conducted,...preliminary findings from animal and laboratory studies suggest that a chemical found in turmeric-called curcumin- may have anti-inflammatory and anticancer properties, but these findings have not been confirmed in people.**"

So what to make from these two conflicting conclusions? Are we to consume turmeric every day?

The honest, sensible assumption about the therapeutic properties of turmeric is that we don't know, but since it has no side effects, tastes good and is not very expensive, it should be a welcome addition to our diet.

Cranberry has been traditionally recommended to treat existing urinary tract infections and garlic to control blood pressure, lower cholesterol, slow the development of atherosclerosis and lower the risk of certain cancers, but according to the NIH, these claims are unproven but permissible.

Scientists in their investigations reported mixed results regarding green tea's ability to either protect against cancer, reduce weight and/or lower blood cholesterol from its antioxidant properties.

To be more emphatic: there are many commonly used spices that perhaps may have a beneficial action. Since they are tasty, relatively cheap and accessible with no side effects, their use should be supported, keeping in mind that the final scientific proof has not yet been determined.

Others are a different story: herbs like Saw palmetto, which is sold by the millions to reduce the size of the prostate, had never been shown scientifically to be effective; when the popular St. John's Wort was put to the test for treating mild to moderate depression, the herb was no more effective than a placebo in two large well-designed studies. Similarly, there are thousands of herbal compounds that are useless.

Some herbs or natural substances exert a negative interaction with prescription medications; for example, fish oil enhances the potency of Coumadin, an anticoagulant, and by doing so it can trigger bleeding in the brain.

An alternative to taking medicinal herbs is to eat fresh fruits and vegetables with proven anti-inflammatory properties, boosting the immune system and limiting the proliferation of vessels (angiogenesis), a permissive factor for tumors to grow and expand.

To sum it up, herbs contained in food, teas, or liquids are desirable, while herbs sold in specialty stores should be consumed with caution if at all since they are expensive and generally useless.

The NIH and other NGOs are sponsoring studies to assess the benefits of herbs and alternative or complementary methods to treat disease because there is a legitimate preoccupation with the **overconsumption of prescription medications,** which have serious side effects, many serious and others lethal. A thorough explanation of the medication culture is found in Chapter 7.

11

Steroids, Hormones and sports drinks enhance physical performance. But...

Athletes have been taking illegal drugs to increase their physical performance for years. Marion Jones, the Olympic champion sprinter, recently acknowledged the use of THG or tetrahydrogestrinone, a powerful anabolic steroid, during the Sydney Olympics, where she won three gold and two bronze medals. As a result, the IOC nullified the relay results. Endurance medications, as they are also known, are effective in muscle building and reducing fat, decreasing fatigue, improving stamina or stopping the pain associated with a physical effort. This class of medications is legitimately used by physicians for the treatment of delayed puberty and wasting conditions like cancer and AIDS; they are effective for children of short stature, stimulating bone growth. Used at the proper dose and under medical supervision, they are effective and side effects can be arrested or avoided. Modified anabolic steroids are administered by physicians to some elderly patients with the purpose of delaying the aging process, at a proper dose and for a limited period of time. In these contexts their use is acceptable, but in sports it is illegal because they give an artificial advantage and because, if unchecked, they have serious collateral effects.

Since these substances are banned for consumption by the general public, the idea of developing an innocuous pill or a drink to improve performance and strength became a highly desirable idea. Nothing of this type exists today, and yet there are many pills and drinks promising to improve stamina, relieve exhaustion and help physical performance. As part of a marketing strategy, they claim to support the immune system, boost health, metabolize fat, give extra energy, cure fatigue, increase mental alertness, enhance physical performance and detoxify the body--claims that have never been substantiated. These assertions are highly deceptive. In the name of freedom of expression and free commerce, these companies are allowed to sell the illusion that we can achieve strength with little effort by taking their products. Who wouldn't want to improve vigor, reboot the body after exercising, and feel strong and tireless just by taking a power drink or popping a pill?

These beverages usually contain caffeine, vitamins, minerals and herbal supplements (like guarana, which also contains caffeine). With the exception of high dose caffeine and illicit drugs, none of the components can boost energy. High doses of caffeine have undesirable side effects like nervousness, stomach upsets, heart arrhythmias and insomnia and have been linked to death in over-performing athletes.

Gatorade is a popular drink that was first introduced to improve the athletic performance of the players of the Gators, the football team at the University of Florida, hence its name. It is an excellent source of water and minerals, which athletes lose through their skin during strenuous exercising and is also used in cases of diarrhea to reestablish water and salt balance. Strenuous physical activity requires fluid, carbohydrate and mineral replacement; in that sense Gatorade and similar beverages are an easy way to provide them, but to believe that they are potent stimulants and can increase strength and improve performance is a delusion.

There are about 110 brands of sport drinks involved in false advertisement; they play in the same league with thousands of other products that resort to gimmicks to create the illusion that they provide something that they don't: vitamins in shampoo that do nothing to your hair, skin creams with concocted 'moisturizers', toothpastes that assure healthier teeth than their competitors, hair nourishment from oat proteins and thousands of others.

Quercetin is a flavonoid found in apple skins, berries, red wine, some vegetables and black tea that was shown to significantly enhance performance … in **mice.** Athletes taking Quercetin perform well but no better than those taking placebos. Some experiments in mice showed that Quercetin may be carcinogenic.

12

This brings us to placebos. In certain situations the results of applying certain treatments, taking certain medications or simply doing things that we believe are helpful in improving our wellbeing are not due to the effects of an active substance but to the power of the mind. The placebo action may be very strong. It influences pain perception, induces muscle relaxation, decreases stress, depression, anxiety and increases physical performance and endurance.

The neurophysiological mechanisms of the brain involved in all body process are well understood in certain areas; for example, we know how the human body responds to physical injury. It does so by putting into action multiple defense and protective mechanisms; for example, raising body temperature, feeling pain and getting an inflammatory response in the area of injury, which is followed by a reparative process. The placebo result is like the response to body harm, an effect that may be understood in the context of an evolved response that protects oneself from a perceived harm. A typical example is a placebo taken for pain, which triggers the perception that the discomfort has lessened. Placebos are also called sugar pills, because traditionally they have been administered as such, but they come in different forms and shapes. A physician in certain contexts is able to help a patient by doing nothing but being there, explained by the influence of an anticipatory response; his presence exerts a placebo effect that may be enhanced just by telling a patient that he/she will be fine. In those circumstances, the doctor is the drug.

The mechanism by which a placebo exerts its effects is believed to result from the release of endogenous opioids, a theory substantiated by the fact that if a patient receives naloxone, an opioid antagonist the placebo effect disappears.

The way the placebo is presented has a strong correlation with the result it renders. The shape and color of a pill that resembles others that were effective in the past is more likely to evoke a positive response. A placebo with a sour taste is more likely to help than a sweet one because traditionally medications are supposed to taste bad. The name of what we consume also has an influence. Names like Boost, Immune Plus, and Shock Therapy to name just a few, suggest a promise that may be fulfilled even if they contain no active ingredients.

A positive placebo response should not be interpreted as an indication that there is no organic or physical basis for a patient's condition, since they may exert a positive result in organic conditions like arthritis, cancer, and other ailments. The following case underscores this statement. Julie, a patient I once saw in consultation, was considered by others to be affected with Irritable Bowel Syndrome, a condition that can be very taxing, has no clinical markers (blood tests, imaging studies and the like) and where the diagnosis is made by patient's manifestations and ruling out organic disease. She, like many patients considered to be functional, was given non-active medications, to exert, in the doctor's mind, a placebo effect. She improved for a while, which seemed to corroborate the diagnosis, but a year later she continued with the same symptomatology; after her work-up she was found to have celiac disease, an organic condition which may be severe in its manifestations and is easily cured by a gluten free diet.

Studies comparing hormone replacement therapy versus placebo for menopause have shown that the placebo effect has astoundingly achieved almost similar results as active drugs. I have gone to a chiropractor to get relief for my back pain from manipulation of my spine. With all the sounds from cracking vertebrae, I felt better, but for no longer than one or two days.

Acupuncture, yoga, homeopathy, herbal therapy, natural remedies, certain techniques or instruments to relieve back pain, non-prescription medications to improve sexual vigor or headaches and spiritual exercises have been the subjects of multiple studies, and all failed to explain the reason for their beneficial effect at a physiological level other than the placebo effect. This should not devaluate or demean the value of a placebo because in the end it may exert a positive response, sometimes better than prescription drugs.

13

The need to be cautious in interpreting scientific data:

The Department of Biology at Boston College is an exemplary institution with a reputable faculty staff dedicated, among other endeavors, to discern the mysteries of certain maladies at a cellular level. They perform research and teaching in genetics, immunology, neuroscience and cell and molecular biology. A research study published in 2007 by members of the staff showed that a calorically restricted diet is an effective alternative to treat malignant brain cancer in mice.

They implanted malignant brain tumors in these animals and divided them in two groups; one received a restricted caloric diet and the other an unrestricted high carbohydrate diet. The first group showed a significantly decreased intracerebral growth of about 35% to 65%. These results are significant and may lead the way to perform clinical studies in patients with this type of cancer.

This and similar studies open the door to the notion that manipulating the content of what we eat, either by caloric intake or composition, may have a dramatic result in curing cancer or avoiding a relapse. David Servan-Schreiber, as we mentioned before, had a brain tumor excised 15 years ago that later recurred. He recommended a diet of fruits and vegetables, which apparently kept the tumor in check for 15 years. He died later from a recurrence. There may be some truth about certain foods producing a good or advantageous effect on different maladies. Fruits and vegetables have antioxidant properties and may boost the immune system; stop the proliferation of vessels, (a prerequisite for tumor growth) or neutralize carcinogenic products.

It is sensible to accept that there is a good way to eat--that fish, fruits and vegetables are good--and a bad way to eat, meaning trans fats, meats and food containing chemicals and artificial additives.

This is far from advocating that diet alone can cure cancer.

14

Lies:

People lie, for financial gain or to satisfy some emotional or psychological or pathological need; lies may be harmless but when it comes to health issues they are dangerous, may produce injury and kill directly or indirectly by delaying a diagnosis, as with the young patient, reported in a previous chapter, who resorted to colon hydrotherapy before seeking medical help and died a year later.

Here are some instances that although preposterous are by no means uncommon; they are so blatant and so obvious that they wouldn't be worth mentioning except that some have become a credo and common practice in some circles.

Dr. Johanna Budwig, a German chemist, was well known for a diet that carried her name. The diet consisted of cottage cheese, flax oil, vegetable juices and other foodstuffs to "cure brain cancer and to prevent or cure other malignancies." She wrote in her book, "The oil-protein shows surprising effect with brain tumors... tumors will be visibly excreted via the throat and nasal passages, perceptible to both patients and caregivers..." this alone is enough to disqualify her. An informed person can easily recognize the false connotation of these claims and yet she had thousands of followers and her book has been a best seller for many years. Even today she has a cadre of devotees that follow her advice and although the diet is harmless, it can be extremely dangerous since patients may forego conventional treatment.

Another blatant lie is the one that advocates special nutrients for curing melanoma, a skin cancer that is invariably fatal if left untreated. Since this condition has a latent period before it manifests with full force, patients who have been promised a cure by nutrition therapy may wrongly believe that they have been restored to health, thus delaying adequate treatment. Melanomas are treated by physicians following a conventional protocol. First they are excised from the skin and if they are superficial, nothing beyond close follow-up is done, other than avoiding sun exposure. If the melanoma is at a more advanced stage, immunotherapy, chemotherapy and/or radiotherapy may be instituted. Delaying treatment usually means delaying potential benefits.

Diet and stress reduction enhance the effectiveness of conventional medical treatment, but it is imperative to be aware of their limitations.

Unscrupulous physicians sometimes administer chemotherapy and radiotherapy in terminal cases to profit financially, with the excuse of offering a last possible hope to terminal patients, knowing quite well that nothing can change a predictable fatal outcome. I have seen patients with terminal pancreatic, liver, colon and other cancers being treated with potent drugs with horrible side effects, increasing their suffering and done solely with the purpose of profiteering.

Here are other lies that twist the truth by utilizing proven facts and distorting them for personal gain:

Acai Berry

That the berry-pulp lowers cholesterol, helps to reduce weight, boosts energy, slows down the antiaging process, improves the digestive health system, and reduces heart disease and cancer risk is part of a fantasy; those claims have never been proven and, as with others, create a world of false illusions. It is a very popular supplement because the fruit is a good source of antioxidants, fiber and heart-healthy fats but it falls short of being a miracle drug.

Laxatives can help in losing weight

Laxatives have been included in many diet supplements surreptitiously or openly to promote weight loss and they do so by removing necessary fluids and electrolytes. Some weight reducing concoctions contain added diuretics and amphetamines, a dangerous cocktail that can lead to irreparable consequences.

The Lemon Diet – The Cabbage Soup Diet- The Morning Banana Diet and the Grapefruit Diet.

These food fads have no scientific basis. The cabbage soup diet made people lose weight because it is restrictive in calories and not because of the cabbage itself, and since it is rich in salt and has little protein, it is unacceptable for the long run; the grapefruit diet, which first appeared in the 30s is still popular among many people who claim that the fruit has the property of burning fat fast, but as with others it is the restriction of calories responsible for reducing weight; the same can be said of the lemon diet. Their adherents assert that it has cleansing properties, eliminating all impurities of the body. The banana diet, according to its proponents, has fiber and pulls calories away before absorption. At one time the banana diet became so popular in Japan that it created a shortage of the fruit.

Calorie restrictive diets are effective but dangerous because they also restrict the intake of essential nutrients like proteins, minerals and vitamins.

In summary:

The above are a miniscule list of thousands of facts, some old, some new, that is part of our universe and has been adopted by many with variable consequences and although most are harmless, others can be deadly.

Processed foods contain too much salt, fat, sugar, chemicals and preservatives, which threatens the homeostasis of the human body. One must be careful replacing food with all kinds of ill-conceived concoctions.

We overuse prescription and over-the-counter medications, are exposed to air pollutants, drink toxins present in water, breathe fumes from vehicles, are exposed to medication errors, undergo unnecessary surgical interventions, use tobacco and recreational drugs, drink excessive alcohol, use cell phones while driving, don't wear seat belts, drive defective cars and use unreliable appliances--all of which are the source of injury, sickness, or death, which explains why in spite of the scientific and technological advances, infirmities are not going away and are actually increasing in frequency.

In the last chapter of this book, I have made a proposition about how to avoid being struck by the noxious elements that are around us.

We all live our lives as if nothing bad is ever going to hit us, until the day that something happens, at which time the first question is always: why me? Sometimes we have an answer. When I had a cardiac arrest in my mid-50s, I wanted to learn why. I was fit and my previous blood tests, including a cholesterol check, were normal. I attributed the event to my strong family history of cardiac disease. Family history is a well-determined factor and yet a vague one, unless we can detect genetic or other markers. In my case there were no definitive biological indicators. Digging further, I came to the conclusion that a threat of a malpractice suit that never materialized had me under uncontrollable stress, which I swept under the carpet to be able to continue with my daily activities. I am convinced that had I confronted the circumstances that I was going through, I probably could have avoided the occurrence. I had a narrowing of the left circumflex coronary artery, likely the factor that initiated the event, but it was an aggregated, persistent vasospasm at that level, triggered by stress, which precipitated the incidence.

Alex was 55 years old when he contracted Multiple Myeloma, a hematological cancer that is invariably fatal. He was married with three children, a cheerful and easygoing individual known by his friends to be a unique storyteller. He mentioned that he was not taking medications and that a physical checkup one year before was normal. When he got sick he also asked the perpetual question: why me? I tried to give him an answer. Alex had a rewarding job, lived in a happy family environment, had no obvious stress, was not a smoker, was not overweight and his diet consisted of typical American food. The more I learned about his daily routine, family history, his personality and other factors, the more I realized that I could not give him an adequate answer. He did not have any known risks factors and in my mind to tell him 'stuff happens' was unacceptable. He was one of the 40 percent of Americans who will contract some kind of cancer during their lifetime.

Is it something we drink, or eat; bisphenol A or phthalate, chemicals used to soften plastics of plastic containers; fertilizers present in food; high radon levels in the household(a source of radiation linked to cancer); air pollutants from car gas emissions; an unknown bacteria or virus; radiation from excessive exposure to X-rays or CAT scans; chemical compounds used in manufacturing building materials; or triclosan (an antibacterial agent which is a common ingredient in soaps and deodorants) responsible for generating a malignancy?

The answer to the cancer dilemma is not at hand yet, but today, with all available data, is it is fair to advance the theory that a combination of external agents in a susceptible individual is responsible for making us sick.

There is hope that we can be active in changing what we do and thereby avoid infirmities.

Stopping tobacco and recreational drugs, avoiding infections and ionizing and ultraviolet light, minimizing occupational hazards, avoiding pollution and radiation exposure and a diet rich in fiber and antioxidants are all essential in maintaining wellness. Adding routine exercise, avoiding stress and having knowledge of our genetic makeup and family history will add quality years to our lives.

These are both simple and complicated undertakings, but you can do it.

Chapter 4:

The Nutrition Corollary – Part 4

"To eat is a necessity, but to eat intelligently is an art." -La Rochefoucauld

What we eat lays the foundation for our health. A simplistic but accurate analogy is equating nutrients with the materials used in building a home; if they are defective the flaws may show over time: the house may not be able to sustain the effects of an earthquake, a flood, the rigors of weather, attack by termites and the corrosion of time. If the fabric of our body is not reliable, we may not be able to stay in good shape and may give way to noxious external factors, be unable to fight infections, have our immune system compromised and get sick. The same way that the pipes of a house become rusty and clogged from exposure to caustics or acids our arteries, metaphorically, our pipes will become hard from excessive cholesterol or calcium.

The list of harmful nutrients is short: too much salt, too much fat, too much sugar. This is so simple that it is mind boggling that we are still in the quagmire of poor health.

We live in a free society where anything goes. Food is readily accessible at reasonable prices; its availability, abundance, taste and the indoctrination from the food industry shapes what and how much we eat.

Industrialized, commercial, processed food is bad because of its content; it is the silent aggressor that, given enough time, will make us sick. The food industry, with its pervasive and relentless actions, has replaced simple, organic, natural and pure basic foods with unhealthy edibles.

In our quest to stay physically fit we are exposed to the merchants of hope selling fad diet books, appetite suppressants and other paraphernalia, and we fall for them because it is an easy, albeit false or dangerous, path to lose weight.

In previous chapters we uncovered deceiving, untrusting and devious practices and have recognized the hurdles to staying in good health. It is the combination of many factors that makes the road to health so difficult. Our body fails by being tempted by nutrients that others want us to consume so they can make a financial profit.

You may ask yourself after reading the previous chapters if I am exposing a conspiracy of sorts aimed to slowly make us sick. It is therefore pertinent at this time for me to be clear one more time about the purpose of this book, since you will ask the same question after reading the chapters on the medical profession and the drug industry. I don't believe that a group of people have purposely designed secret plans to commit illegal acts to make us sick, but I am convinced that in the process of commercialization they have succumbed to the temptation of making easy money with a blatant disregard for our wellbeing. The history of tobacco companies clearly illustrates how sound commercial practices are replaced by devious actions aimed to protect financial gains. When after several centuries nicotine proved without equivocation to be addictive and a significant health hazard, the manufacturers strongly denied those facts; only when legal action was taken against them did they come to terms with reality. The immorality of selling a product that causes cancer, respiratory and cardiovascular disease is obvious and does not deserve discussion. Sometimes corporations caught in fraudulent activities pay civil penalties, which amount to a small proportion of their gains. Make a billion, settle for a million in fines, case closed.

I have exposed devious practices to give you the tools to stay away from what may harm you. You may have taken pleasure in reading the different stories described in this book or identify with some of them because you or somebody you know may have lived similar experiences. If that is all you have internalized, I would not have accomplished my goal. You need to feel the anger and mobilize your rage to do what is right, that is, stop patronizing those who are maiming us in a slow, pervasive, and relentless way. When myths are metaphorical they don't hurt; deceptions and lies do.

Since life is about decisions, it is time to outline a plan to eat well. By choosing the right stuff, you will stay healthy, strong and vigorous. Your wellbeing starts with what you eat--a difficult and yet simple task. It is hard to believe that we are in a state of affairs where 66 percent of us are overweight and that we get sick from what we consume.

With knowledge comes responsibility. Now that we have learned the facts and untangled the lies, it is time to walk the road to health.

The first step is to outline a strategy to make sure that our bones, heart, muscles and the rest of our infrastructure is in optimal shape; this will assure that bodily functions will not be compromised. The different systems of the human body have a threshold for tolerating injury that comes in the form of inflammation, degenerative changes and cancer. For instance and to be more graphic, excessive fat in the blood on a constant basis overwhelms its metabolic pathway and it deposits surplus on the walls of the arteries, altering the flow of blood that in many cases leads to heart, brain or liver dysfunction. Other organs may fail as well; cancer of the prostate may arise from eating too much fat; too much salt is a source of high blood pressure; lack of calcium produces osteoporosis. In other words, the quality and amount of all nutrients is the mainstay for a healthy body and strong function.

The following is a common sense plan:

The first step is to know your body mass index (BMI), a measure of weight in relation to height.

> Underweight: BMI less than 18.5
> Normal: 18.5-24.9
> Overweight: 25.9-29.9
> Obese: 30 and above
> Morbidly Obese: 40 and above

Underweight, obese and morbidly obesity are pathological conditions, not ifs or buts and they require immediate intervention.

Weight alone is not the only factor that produces disease. There are external agents, inborn errors of metabolism, genetics, family predisposition, immunity and low defense mechanisms that may trigger an ailment, but even under that circumstance, excess weight will make a person more vulnerable. Those who are in a good state of nutrition and physically fit prevent and fight disease better.

A basal check-up by a physician is mandatory, independent of symptoms. For people with no obvious medical problems, the recommendation is to visit an internist once a year. A diagnosis of normalcy is one more reason to adhere to a healthy diet. Don't get fooled if your doctor tells that everything is perfect; if **you are overweight**, even if your tests and physical examination are normal **today,** you need to shed those extra pounds to avoid future damage to your body.

In addition to knowing your BMI, it is important to **measure waist circumference** because it serves as a predictor of heart disease, hypertension and diabetes. Doctors seldom measure a patient's waist, a simple test that only requires a measuring tape.

Establish your goals:

If you are normal your goal should be to remain fit and healthy by eating well and exercising on a regular basis

If you are a large person who is **mildly** overweight, have healthy eating habits, exercise regularly and feel good with the way you look, you may not need to shed pounds, providing you don't have obesity-associated conditions. This will remove the anxiety and undue preoccupation that usually comes with the effort to lose weight, yet it is vital to get periodic checkups for early detection of disease. Being satisfied with your health gives a sense of confidence and optimism and a valued image of your persona.

If you are **morbidly obese** you need to work to move the dial of the scale down, even if you have no symptoms or visible medical problems. Denial is life threatening. **Today's healthy obese is tomorrow's sick person because the damage is cumulative and the consequences appear at a later time.**

Once the goals have been established it is time to set a timetable. Crash diets are undesirable because invariably you will abandon the effort and end up in failure. Conversely, shedding pounds slowly creates a habit, a way of eating and a sensible approach that has a better chance of becoming a permanent habit. Dieting needs to be done in a context where guilt or shame has no place. There are lots of circumstances blocking your good intentions. Temptation to eat hypercaloric and tasty, although harmful, food is everywhere; in previous chapters we have identified the enemy. It is time to fight. This is not a metaphor. Too much food today will do harm at the end of a long encounter.

And, don't fool yourself thinking that just by exercising you can forgo adhering to a sensible diet. The road to health does not admit equivocations.

Review your armamentarium:

 Before starting on any type of diet, understanding that it is a hard and difficult task, you should review the instruments available to fight the fight.

You may decide that you can do it on your own, or choose to join other people with similar problems who meet regularly to discuss how to achieve the same goal, or seek professional help.

A support group provides needed psychosocial benefits. Sharing stories and experiences with other people provides an incentive to do what others have done to achieve success. A network of obese patients is similar to other groups with other habits like alcohol and drugs, where getting together allows for identification with others and an understanding that you are not alone in a deleterious predicament.

The entire household needs to become involved in the process of weight loss. This should be approached as a team effort. It is easy for the affected individual to succumb to the temptations of a refrigerator or pantry stuffed with tempting edibles, like ice cream, cookies, pastries, sweets, jelly beans, chocolate, snacks, butter, whole milk, and others. The way to get rid of this conundrum is to make everybody in the home decide which foodstuffs are permissible and which are not. For instance, chocolate could be permitted since it is tasty and has antioxidant properties, providing that one limits the intake to no more than a set amount. Corn chips should not, red wine is acceptable, vegetables and fruit should be at hand to satiate your appetite, refined sugars should be avoided and saturated fats should be thrown out the window.

Review your routine; don't patronize restaurants that may serve luscious food full of calories. A nacho platter contains 900 calories, a cone of ice cream from 600 to 900, and one portion of chocolate cake 600. These three items alone fulfill your daily requirements and contain for the most part unwanted, empty calories.

Before you start this quest for health, be aware that it is going to be a hard-fought war. You will be tempted to retreat, you will find excuses not to do it, you will invoke being under stress, or busy, or in places where is difficult to get healthy foods, or in social gatherings where food is abundant. Excuses are easy to come by, but your commitment should prevail.

The odds have not been in your favor in the past, but by achieving sensible and practical goals and by setting your expectations to a realistic level, you will win the obesity war. Not that you cannot occasionally eat a hypercaloric meal, but it should be done within certain limits. Eat slowly and you will savor your food better than if you gulp. Today is your birthday and you want to eat a steak: just go ahead, but remove the fat, leave a little bit on your plate and avoid hypercaloric side dishes. If you are in a restaurant, don't make the bread basket disappear before they bring the main course. Two pieces of bread and butter may give you 500 hundred unwanted extra calories. Don't fall for appetite suppressants, diet books, hypnosis and other fads. It is you who should be in control and not be controlled by others.

The War Plan:

Eating the right stuff and avoiding the wrong stuff is so simple that it is incredible that we are still in this quandary. We need a cultural transformation to facilitate lifestyle modification.

The obstacles are coming from the food industry, fast food eateries, newly developed artificial agricultural practices and misinformation. They have changed our way of life for the worse. I suspect that we were better off in the past when the milk was coming directly from the cow and the produce from small farms. Anyway, that was then and this is now. These are the new rules:

Read it carefully:

Rule 1: Do not eat processed food.

Rule 2: Avoid salty food, saturated fat and fatty foods.

Rule 3: Eat three times a day and a snack like fruit or vegetables.

Rule 4: Eat slowly, chew well (the digestive process starts in your mouth).

Rule 5: Moderate amounts of red wine, occasional beer and occasional liqueur are permissible.

Rule 6: Olive and canola oil and non-saturated fats are encouraged.

Rule 7: Forget about soft drinks; they have no nutritional value, are fattening and are loaded with sugar.

Rule 8: Refined sugars like the one found in cakes, pasta, white bread and potatoes should be used sparingly because they have little nutritional value.

Rule 9: Eat from smaller plates.

Rule 10: Cook your own food; you will get pleasure in becoming the chef of the house.

Rule 11: Animals are the enemy, plants are your friends.

Rule 12: Changing eating habits is a long-term commitment; quick fixes don't work.

Rule 13: Variation of ingredients and in cooking is a key to success

Rule 14: Eat when you are hungry, not when you are depressed, bored or upset.

The ideal diet should contain protein, carbohydrates and proteins in different degrees, minerals, vitamins and fiber; which takes us to:

Rule 15: A healthy diet is easy to define and consists of the liberal intake of fruits, legumes and vegetables, grains, nuts and dairy.

This should be the base of any diet to which very little beef, poultry, eggs and butter. Fish may be added.

Make sure that what you consume is organic, not processed or with added chemicals or additives. Eat only seasonal food. Try to eat local foods, those that have been grown on neighborhood farms or in your own garden. It requires effort and patience to learn where to buy them but it is fun; there is a certain collegiality among people that go to the farmers market because they share a sense of purpose. Find farmers market or fresh food specialty stores in your neighborhood. Be suspicious of good looking fruits or vegetables with no aroma since they are usually chemically treated. Don't be fooled by labels, reduced fat does not mean healthy since it may contain no nourishing ingredients. Antioxidants are contained in different foods in the form of vitamins, minerals, carotenoids and polyphenols and they are good because they have anti-inflammatory properties, may slow the degenerative process by slowing oxidative stress (a normal body function), reduce (not eliminate) the risk of cancer, retard the appearance of Alzheimer's disease, and protect cardiovascular function. We are in the early stages in understanding the value of antioxidant which may affect health through gene-nutrient interaction.

Variety assures easier compliance; eating the same thing over and over again is boring and triggers failure.

Social, cultural and economic considerations are important in adjusting to a diet plan. When I moved to the US in 1975 I used to visit my mother twice a year in Buenos Aires. We invariably shared a meal with my siblings, like old times. She would serve puchero (a stew of chicken, potatoes, carrots, cabbage, pumpkin and corn on the cob, to be smashed and dressed with large amount of oil and plenty of salt, of course), milanesa (breaded veal cutlet) with fries, cheese blintzes, to name a few of the hypercaloric, remarkably tasty foods. She would not accept any excuse to leave something on our plate. Since I only visited few days, that was OK. There is nothing wrong in not obsessing about what we eat. Mother was happy and we all were satisfied physically and emotionally.

Fish, rich in Omega oil, is a valuable addition to any diet, providing it is not contaminated with noxious chemicals. Salmon, trout and herring are rich in good quality proteins.

Deep frying is an unhealthy cooking habit. Deep fried chicken tastes good but contains unhealthy saturated fats. Always use vegetable, not animal, oil. The latter contains noxious fatty acids.

Adjust your daily intake of calories to your individual needs, your body frame and the amount of energy you expend.

Diets high in fruits, legumes and vegetables with moderate amounts of dietary fiber may reduce or prevent the incidence of chronic diseases and although the evidence is not 100 percent conclusive yet, the understating of their nutritional value suggests that they are the preferred edibles; the recommendation is to include at least five servings of fruit and vegetables a day and include large amounts of cereal grains.

READ THESE 15 RULES AGAIN AND AGAIN UNTIL THEY BECOME SECOND NATURE.

A note about Nutrition:

Diets are difficult to adhere to. Eating well is a long term investment in good health. Follow simple principles; avoid magical solutions because they do not exist. Don't try an easy way out because you will be wasting time and money. Be suspicious of those offerings presented as the *last* diet that you will ever need to follow.

Watch out for the scammers and the unscrupulous big corporations interested in their profits and not your health. Be aware of the obstacles on the road to good health.

Organic, natural, unprocessed, unrefined food, with little fat and little salt, is the name of the game. Food treated by a chemical or industrial process is the adversary. Just go back to page 98 and read the composition of the burger bun and you will understand why.

If you cannot accomplish your intentions on your own, ask for help. Social workers, dietitians, physicians, weight control centers, and health clinics are there to help. It is your life.

Nutrisystem, Weight Watchers, The Zone and others provide low calorie, well balanced, restaurant type edibles, which helps in shedding excessive weight; understanding that it is a **temporary tool** that you may use to achieve an acceptable weight, after which time your own kitchen should take over.

There are more drastic measures available in the firmament of weight loss like Bariatric surgery. These procedures are usually performed laparoscopically and cause significant weight loss, while at the same time improving or correcting diabetes, hypertension and reducing mortality rate in general. It is recommended for obese people with a body mass index of 40 or more who have failed conventional treatments and have co-morbid conditions. It is remarkable that these high risk patients go home one or two days after this major surgical procedure. About 20 percent of patients may experience transient post-surgical complications. Mortality is very low providing the surgery is performed by experienced surgeons in specialized medical centers. A longitudinal study published in 2009 in the NEJM showed a mortality rate of 0.3 percent, contradicting another study by David Arteburn, published in October 2009 in the *Archives of Surgery,* which showed a mortality rate of 6.3 percent in a group of 856 individuals with a mean age of 54 who underwent the operation. This is one of the few studies that have followed patients for such a long period of time. **The operation is not without morbid complications or death and therefore should be used only when every noninvasive method fails and mainly when associated morbid conditions linked to obesity become more dangerous than the operation itself.**

An important and final note about Nutrition

Diets have failed people again and again. Only 2 to 4% of persons that have engaged on a diet are able to keep their weight down. Diets, programs, systems and most plans to lose weight are effective, providing one can adhere to them forever, and that is impossible and implausible. Therefore they should be substituted by a permanent way of eating a high quality, proper quantity of foodstuffs.

There are biological, cultural, psychological, social and physical reasons that trigger obesity, as we explained in previous chapters, and unless we attack all those aspects, we will not succeed in achieving sensible weight loss.

The only way to lose weight and keep it off is to change your mindset and your approach to the task of becoming healthy. You already know or have learned from previous chapters which are the desirable and the undesirable foodstuffs. **But nothing is prohibited**. Pasta and simple sugars have a high glycemic index (or how long it takes to raise the blood sugar) therefore you should eat them only sporadically and the same with meats and animal products. You already know that there are bad and good carbs, that saturated and trans fats are very bad, that colorful fruits and vegetables are great, that whole grain breads are excellent, as well as oats, and that beans are very nutritious because they contain good quality protein. Other high protein vegetables like Brussels sprouts, lentils, couscous, almonds, and wheat gluten can substitute for meat.

Since you already know all this, it only takes adjusting the portions of the good quality food and you are set. Eating well then becomes second nature--**no guilt trips anymore**, **no anxiety** about eating a non-desirable item once in a while. Eat when you are hungry and don't eat when you are not hungry. Be creative, combine 'the good guys' in such a way that they will become palatable, exquisite if you wish. You don't need diet books; you need cookbooks or cooking lessons. It is fun, it is good, and it is inspirational. Trust me; you will feel full eating exactly the right amount of calories and the right nutrients.

In the next chapters you will learn the other factors that influence our wellbeing, and once we learn to tackle them, we will be on our way to achieving optimal health.

Chapter 5:

PHYSICAL FITNESS

The importance of being fit

Physical fitness is not only one of the most important keys to a healthy body; it is the basis of a dynamic and creative intellectual activity.-John F. Kennedy

1

Combining healthy eating with sound and judicious exercise provides two pillars for achieving strength and vigor. Fitness increases heart and lung performance, adds flexibility of the body and enhances stamina.

Metabolic conditions like diabetes may reverse with dieting and exercise. Hypertension may be controlled without medications, osteoporosis may be halted and overall the quality of life improves.

When I was a kid growing in Buenos Aires, we had one hour of physical education a week in school. There were no programmed sport activities. I used to play soccer with my friends *en el barrio,* but I was such a bad player that seldom was I invited back. My mother did not have too much understanding about the importance of sports and physical activities; I was called el 'gordito' (the fat one) for a long time. Physical fitness and staying in shape was not an everyday concern. Only sophisticated parents would encourage their kids to exercise. Sports were mainly recreational and not practiced with the aim of staying healthy or losing weight. Jogging did not exist; if you saw somebody running in the street you thought that he was running away from the police--even the word jogging had to be borrowed from the English language. People did not walk with the purpose of working out, only to go from here to there. When jogging in Buenos Aires caught up with the rest of the world, it became a new craze that persists until today. Argentineans are very creative; when I visited in the early 1980s my friends invited me to join them in one of their daily jogging session. This was a group of 20 acquaintances that run together from 6:30 to 8 o'clock in the evening in Los bosques de Palermo (Palermo Woods), a setting similar to Central Park, a vast green area with artificial lakes and a huge variety of trees and multiple areas of recreation. Twice a week after jogging, everybody brought one meal and wine for a picnic as a reward for their efforts. Camaraderie made running tolerable and pleasurable.

There were many athletic clubs aimed more at social gatherings than promoting physical fitness. The culture of sports was directed to entertain. Players were players for the love of the game and not for financial remuneration. Soccer is the national sport and Argentina is a powerful team in all World Cups. Equestrianism, polo, rugby, tennis, golf, skiing, fencing and swimming were practiced mainly by the elites for leisure and enjoyment, not as part of a fitness curriculum. Bodybuilding was the terrain mainly of narcissistic individuals with aesthetic aspirations without consideration of health. Gymnastics, calisthenics, jumping, sprinting were practiced by amateurs mainly for competition purposes and not remuneration.

In the early fifties the majority of the population was not preoccupied with physical fitness, since little was known about the link of sedentary life and cholesterol, triglycerides, hypertension, the risk of stroke and cardiovascular disease and others. Yet the people in Argentina were not sedentary. Walking to work or to school was common, albeit not intended to exercise. Transportation was not that accessible and cars were expensive, so it was not unusual to walk one or two miles every day. The population of workers performing manual tasks was large and exceeded by far that of deskbound occupations. Combine all this with healthy eating habits, and decades ago obesity was not a problem, similar to what happens in underdeveloped countries. In contrast conditions like obesity, diabetes and hypertension are common in industrialized societies and are labeled as diseases of affluence.

When I arrived in the United States for my training in 1959, I found that the students in school and college were engaged in sports mainly for recreation and competition and exceptional athletes were granted scholarships and were recruited by the best educational institutions. Only in America! Basketball, football, baseball, hockey and skates became my 'new sports'. In every Olympic competition the US was ahead of every other country in gold medals as a testimony to their dedication, commitment and devotion to sports.

The concept of body weight and fitness became a concern among the medical profession when several papers were published showing a link between a sedentary lifestyle and disease and the reversal of disease by physical activity. During my rotating internship at Washington Hospital Center, none of my professors taught us the benefits of physical activity as we know it today or the link between inactivity and disease.

We learned–starting in the sixties–that sedentary people were more likely to die earlier than their counterparts and as a result, exercising became part of the heath paradigm. Gyms proliferated; people of all ages increased their physical activity; walking, jogging and running are today part of the landscape; use it or lose it became a nice catch-phrase applied to physical condition, brain function, sex and other activities. The physical trainer stopped being a rarity. Health clubs became more sophisticated, offering all forms of training. Pilates (invented by Joseph Pilates in the early twentieth century) exploded as a way of physical training in the last three decades. Its name stopped being proprietary and today anybody, trained or untrained, qualified or not ,can offer Pilates, or something that looks like it, to the public. Spinning, a high intensity bicycling exercise first developed in the 80s, became a popular endeavor. New equipment and machinery was invented to cure back pain, diminish abdominal girth, increase muscle mass and augment joint motion or to allow people to exercise painlessly, clearly an oxymoron.

There is universal consensus that exercise is part of a healthy lifestyle, and yet **40 percent of the people in the United States are sedentary.**

Advice to engage in physical activities is being accepted better than nutritional recommendations. People who pay a monthly fee to join a gym don't want to see their money wasted, which becomes an incentive to attend. Exercise, if done seriously, is hardly recreational and not effortless; it takes endurance to walk on a treadmill or pedal a stationary bike, but at the end the release of internal endorphins gives a pleasurable sensation that makes the endeavor tolerable and, in contrast to dieting, provides instant gratification. Sweating and struggling boosts our self image; no pain no gain becomes a dictum that serves us well.

2

Why exercise?

There are myriads of scientific papers dealing with the effects of exercise in providing a definitive health benefit. But before we get into the subject, let me preface it with these comments for a better understanding.

The process of reaching a valid scientific assumption is multifaceted. For example, to learn if people affected with essential hypertension might be able to reverse the condition by exercising alone and without medication, it is necessary to conduct a randomized, double blind placebo controlled investigation. This is usually achieved by the unsystematic allocation of patients in two groups, one of which will receive the purported treatment and the other a placebo. The number of patients needs to be large enough to avoid occasional variations, and the results have to be statistically significant. To avoid bias, the experiment needs to be 'double blind,' meaning that neither the patient nor the investigator would know what the patient is taking. In medicine these types of trials are considered to be the most reliable way of learning about the benefits or problems associated with a medication or a procedure. In the case of exercising, comparative studies become more difficult because it is hard to find a placebo to simulate a physical activity. Another way to assess the value of certain treatments and/or procedures is by utilizing what is called evidence-based medicine. This is a method that seeks to measure benefits and risks of certain medical decisions that allow us to predict outcomes based on science. This is an important advance in medicine because it allows us to support what we do in everyday practice.

For example, when a patient arrives in the emergency room with chest pain and there is a suspicion that he/she may be having a heart attack, we administer aspirin to prevent platelet aggregation, which minimizes the blockage in a coronary artery. We do this before we have total substantiation that a heart attack is ensuing.

Which brings us to our topic: **based on science, it is safe to say that being in good physical shape prolongs life, gives a state of wellbeing and halts or reverses many medical conditions**. This conclusion is the result of multiple well-designed investigations.

A generalized observation is that people who exercise three times a week appear to be healthy and have a sense of wellbeing not present in sedentary people.

Training enhances physical activity; practicing sports and fitness exercises increases self esteem. Exercising requires persistence, commitment and effort. Working out gives peoples a sense of achievement and comfort. This appears to be related to the release of endorphins in the brain, which produces mood enhancement and alleviates mental and physical pain. This morphine-like substance blocks pain pathways.

Children who engage in sports are less likely to use drugs, alcohol or commit crimes. Alejandro Gutman, an ex-soccer player and current owner of a syndicated sport radio program, created a plan for children from El Salvador, that he called Futbol Forever, which consists mainly of the practice of specific exercises that slowly help them connect to their emotional and mental development (currently more than 1000 young people are part of this endeavor). The participants are underprivileged children between the ages of 6 and 16. A recent evaluation showed an important impact in their lives. They have improved their behavior in relation to themselves and others, have better performance at school, have enhanced their self confidence, watch less television and have improved reflection. Since the inception of this curriculum, there has been a decline in violence and crime. Kids became more expressive, communicative and sociable and the impact in their everyday life has been astonishing, creating a life with a purpose.

The payback of physical activity does not stop there. There is a wealth of evidence that physical activity enhances bone mass and strength and is beneficial in all stages of life.

There is not one single defined set of physical activities to promote bone strength, but rather a host of programs adjusted to sex, age and maturity or fragility of the population. Scans and MRIs have shown the specific geometric, structural and microstructural bone properties that adapt to weight bearing activity, creating stronger bones.

Drs. Laurie Barclay and Desiree Lie, in *Medscape,* cited a longitudinal, prospective, observational cohort study of men in the so-called Uppsala study during a 35 year period to examine the association between physical exercise and mortality rates. It showed that high and medium physical activity was associated with lower mortality rates in men 50 years or older and that the effect of increasing physical activity from low to high levels or from medium to high levels between the ages of 50 and 80 years was similar to smoking cessation, with a health risk reduction of 10 years in those with high physical activity.

The same authors in another article highlighted the benefits of physical activity and exercise. These effects are significant and as such will be transcribed almost verbatim to round out our discussion:

> *Vigorous, long term participation in aerobic exercise training (AET) improves cardiovascular reserve and skeletal muscle adaptation.*
> *Prolonged AET may also reduce age-related accumulation of central body fat, thereby by protecting the heart.*
>
> *Prolonged participation in resistance exercise training (RET) increases muscle and bone mass and strength to a greater extent than AET.*
> *In healthy middle–aged and older adults, three months or more of moderate intensity AET are associated with cardiovascular adaptations which are apparent both at rest and in response to acute dynamic exercise.*
>
> *Beneficial metabolic changes associated with AET include improved glycemic control and clearance of postprandial lipids, as well as preferential utilization of fat during submaximal exercise.*
> *In postmenopausal women, AET may counteract age related decreases in bone mineral density.*
>
> *RET may markedly increase strength and muscular power in older adults.*
>
> *Older and younger adults have similar age related increases in muscle quality and these increases do not appear to be sex specific.*
> *Although the effect of exercise on physical function is poorly understood and may not be linear, RET may improve walking, chair stand, and balance activities.*
>
> *Older adults who regularly take part in moderate or high intensity RET may have increased fat-free mass, decrease total body fat mass and other beneficial changes in body composition.*

In populations at increased risk of falling, multimodal exercise, including strength and balance exercises and tai chi may decrease the risk of noninjurious and sometimes injurious falls.

Regular exercise and physical activity are linked to significant improvement in overall psychological well being, possibly via effects on self-concept and self-esteem.

Physical fitness and AET are linked to a lower risk for clinical depression or anxiety.

Cardiovascular fitness and higher levels of physical activity lower the risk for cognitive decline and dementia.

AET and RET alone or specially combined, improve some measures of cognitive functioning, especially those requiring executive control, in previously sedentary older adults.

High-intensity RET is effective in treating clinical depression.

There are multiple studies in children demonstrating that exercise improves cardiovascular risk factors in children with Type 1 diabetes, reduces obesity, improves motor skills and decreases TV viewing. Fatigue, depression, and anxiety can be effectively controlled or diminished by exercising on a regular basis. Overall, it provides a sense of happiness derived from a combination of factors, including chemical, hormonal, structural, and psychological effects. Self-esteem goes up when body image improves.

3

Which exercise? A common question, a complex answer

Walking is a form of workout; so is climbing or a trapeze used in acrobatics, to mention only three of the hundreds of modalities for physical performance. Once the reader has accepted the premise that being active promotes physical and mental well-being he/she needs to choose one or more modalities to meet his/her goals.

The observation is clear; people who practice some kind of physical activity stay fit and healthier than their counterparts. It is better to engage in a specific type of activity based on individual needs. Some may benefit more from aerobic exercise than resistance training and vice versa. Unless they are under a supervised program, like in a rehabilitation center, or have the advantage of counseling by a certified trainer they may chose to do what comes easy or what their instincts or knowledge or bias tell them to do but not without counseling by a physician, a knowledgeable friend or some trusty acquaintance. Performing the same type of exercise over and over again renders the effort fruitless, although it is better than being inactive. Exercise needs to be performed with caution. Jogging or walking is a popular, worthy form of physical activity and does not require any special equipment other than a comfortable pair of walking shoes and yet even if done properly is not exempt from associated problems. Running injuries are multiple and some of them are serious, requiring medical intervention. Ankle sprain, blisters, foot problems, bloody nipple discharge from the breast, stress fractures and plantar fasciitis are some of the problems connected with jogging.

Knowledge of all the facts surrounding physical activity is indispensable before embarking on any of the hundreds of available exercise alternatives. It is important to comprehend the dynamics and problems associated with a defined type of exercise.

There are two types of exercises: **aerobic exercise training (AET) and resistance exercise training (RET).**

Aerobic training increases respiration and heart rate and provides muscles and tissues with oxygen, which in turn promotes weight loss and increases physical endurance. This is obtained by oxygen getting into the muscles to burn fat and carbohydrates. Think about aerobics as a machine that eliminates fat from the body as efficiently as liposuction, but in a physiological way and without side effects. With regular training the heart starts pumping more blood with each beat and each contraction of the heart becomes more efficient, which explains why athletes have a low resting pulse. Instead of 80 beats a minute the same delivery of oxygen may be achieved with 48 beats. More oxygen means better enzymatic function, better oxygenation and mitochondrial augmentation in number and function (mitochondria is among others the source for chemical energy and cell growth), which makes burning of carbohydrates and fat more efficient.

Aerobic exercise includes running, jogging, treadmill, dancing, elliptical machine, stationary bike and others, any of which can turn into anaerobic (meaning without oxygen) if performed beyond the capability of one's body. Running at a reasonable pace is aerobic but brisk running that makes the individual short of breath exhausts the possibility of obtaining needed oxygen and to compensate the respiratory rate goes up and the accessory muscles involved in breathing work at full capacity.

Aerobic exercise needs to be tailored to physical status. It is important to ask your doctor about possible problems associated with your choice. For example if a person has a knee problem it is better to avoid the impact from a treadmill and use an elliptical machine which has less bearing on the joints.

Patients affected with cardiovascular or pulmonary conditions need special advice, preferably from a rehabilitation center. Physical training needs to be adjusted to age, sex, medical condition, physical status to achieve a definitive goal.

Dr. Mary M. McDermott in the *Journal of the American Medical Association* reported that patients with Peripheral Artery Disease (PAD) with or without intermittent claudication can benefit from regular supervised treadmill exercise and resistance training that targets their lower extremities. This may be counterintuitive because many of these patients fear pain and weakness in the lower limbs. Yet supervised exercise showed an improvement of PAD when compared with a control group.

Resistance Exercise Training is a form of strength training by which the muscles of the body are targeted to improve their mass and consequently, their function. Body builders work on each skeletal muscle, utilizing different targeted machines. The rest of us appear to be content with having a good generalized muscle tone and bone mass.

RET provides the same physical and emotional benefits of AET and they are complementary. RET and AET rely on machines available in most gyms and health clubs.

Running two miles on a treadmill for 30 minutes with an elevation of four burns about 200 calories. The impact on the knees and back may become a problem. A good alternative is to use a stationary bike or an elliptical machine with arm components with the same results regarding the amount of burned calories and cardiopulmonary benefits.

The rowing machine is a machine that uses almost every muscle in the body. It has the advantage of avoiding damage to the knees or other joints with the exception of the back and is very effective in burning calories.

Other pieces of equipment improve the motion and strength of the spine, legs, arms, chest and abdomen. If somebody suffers with back pain, there are specific kinds of training to improve the condition. Big bellies may be corrected by certain workouts that may improve mass of the abdominal muscles but the fat below the skin may not disappear if there is excessive body weight. Strengthening of the abdominal muscles is achieved with simple exercises like pushups and flexion or by using different kinds of equipment aimed at offering different types of resistance to tone and tighten them. **There is a significant correlation between increased abdominal girth and heart ailments, hypertension and possible other ailments.** Of course, we are not talking about a swollen belly that may be a sign of other conditions such as liquid in the belly from liver cirrhosis, cancer or intrinsic abdominal conditions such as intestinal obstruction.

Push-ups strengthen the core muscles, the chest, the shoulders and the triceps. There are specific gymnastics to increase the flexibility, endurance and potency of the body.

In summary, from the plethora of possibilities to work out, you will need to choose the one that is best for you in terms of safety and convenience.

Aerobics directed to improve cardio-respiratory function, combined with resistance training to improve muscle mass and tone, is the most valuable and recommended arrangement. By doing so one achieves maximal return in terms of endurance, cardio-respiratory function, flexibility, increased lean muscle mass, appearance, and self satisfaction

Swimming is one of the best physical exercises that can help people lose weight and stay fit and trim. It has multiple advantages over other physical activities since it has minimal or no deleterious effects on any part of the body, as opposed, for example, to the treadmill that may end up wearing out the knees. In addition, it is an excellent aerobic workout, good for the heart and lungs. It has to be practiced with a plan and an objective. Swimming requires using the right muscles at a set pace in a coordinated way and requires training to avoid converting it into a disorganized, purposeless form of exercise.

Accessories from goggles to leg pulls can help in swimming performance. Different styles of swimming work different muscle groups like the butterfly stroke, back stroke, free style, etc. It is important to master breathing while swimming; good motion and good breathing guarantees maximum benefits. When you walk you are surrounded by air and breathing is unconscious and natural, but in the water breathing is reflexive and voluntary until it becomes mindless and mechanical. Speed of swimming and amount of time spent in this activity depends on your goals.

I am elaborating more about swimming than other exercise because there is scientific evidence that this may be the optimal sport, mainly when it is complemented with resistance exercises for the shoulder, hip, legs and stretching utilizing specific machines.

Swimming is fun and after a while easy to perform correctly. There are private and public health clubs with swimming facilities--for example, there are 2,686 YMCA organizations and most of them have special programs for swimming; only time and dedication is needed. Swimming for one hour burns between 500 and 600 calories, a significant amount.

Alternating between different exercises or sports helps avoid boredom; too much of anything in the end becomes tedious. Avoiding the monotony of engaging in one single set of training exercises has the secondary benefit of keeping other muscle groups active. It is surprising to see people in the gym doing over and over again the same routine when they have available other pieces of equipment that can help achieve flexibility, muscle mass, thoracic expansion, and breathing that one single piece of machine could not do.

Enhanced physical activity, training, gymnastics and sports serve the ultimate purpose of improving voluntary and involuntary body functions. There is no scientific data comparing different kinds of exercise in terms of efficiency, health impact and associated problems. Each method is free terrain to claim that it is the best way to improve stamina, flexibility and cardiopulmonary status when conducted in an organized, systematic way. Comparative studies are not available but there is plenty of information and facts about each individual exercise.

Pilates is one of the most popular forms of exercise and rightly so. It was created by Joseph Pilates, first developed to be practiced on flat surfaces when working with injured soldiers after the First World War. Later he used the springs from their beds to create additional resistance. The idea behind Pilates is to use core muscles to increase the tone of the body, add flexibility, stabilize the spine, prevent or cure back pain and improve posture and balance. Pilates used to be a proprietary name and trainers needed to be certified in order to provide services. Today, after the US Supreme Court ruled that the Pilates name is public domain, anybody can engage as an instructor. **Therefore the reader needs to be cautioned that Pilates is not just a piece of machinery but a serious methodology requiring serious coaching and guidance.**

Tai Chi is a form of martial arts created by the Chinese 2000 years ago and extended to the Occidental civilization, where it is practiced by millions. We all have a fascination for Oriental martial arts since they are intrinsically connected to a philosophical way of life. There is a certain enthrallment in observing groups of people in parks or other spaces moving elegantly and breathing at a rhythmic, musical pace. When I practiced Tai Chi in Pasadena I had a sensation of peace, calm and relaxation that I did not get with any other form of exercise. It improves health and provides an opening for meditation and self defense.

The Mayo Clinic Staff in an article on the Mayo Clinic Proceedings described Tai Chi as meditation in motion. Anyone, regardless of age and physical ability, can practice Tai Chi since it does not require physical prowess. Tai Chi emphasizes technique over strength. It is used to:

Reduce Stress
Increase flexibility
Improve muscle strength and definition
Increase energy, stamina and agility

Increase feelings of wellbeing

It has been a subject of scientific study only in recent years that proved that this discipline, beyond stress reduction, has a multitude of favorable effects, including:

Reduces anxiety and depression Improves balance and coordination Reduces the number of falls. Improves sleep quality, such as staying asleep longer at night and feeling more alert during the day Slows bone loss in women after menopause Lowers blood pressure Improves cardiovascular fitness Relieves chronic pain Improves everyday physical functioning

In August 19, 2010 a leading article published in *The New England of Medicine* showed that Tai chi is an effective alternative treatment for fibromyalgia. Coming from the *NEJM,* the findings need to be taken at face value.

Yoga is another way to improve health, providing it is being practiced routinely and under the supervision of specialized instructors. Yoga originated in India and also has fascinated and permeated into the Occidental civilization, where it is practiced by millions. Yoga traditionally is seen as a means of stress relief but it offers additional health benefits. I am quoting the Mayo Clinic staff from a recently published article about the salutary and useful effects of yoga:

Increases flexibility

Helps in the management of chronic health conditions such as asthma, carpal tunnel syndrome, depression, low back pain, multiple sclerosis, osteoarthritis of the knees and memory problems

> When combined with a vegetarian diet, aerobic exercise and medication, reduces cardiovascular disease rate and blood pressure levels
> Helps weight loss
> Improves balance, and helps to avoid falls and hip fractures.
> People with cancer and their caregivers who practice yoga may improve their quality of life

4

How much exercise is good for you?

It depends on your goal and needs.

Individuals with normal weight are recommended to exercise at least 30 minutes a day. The longer and the harder the exercise, the better results in terms of conditioning heart, lungs and muscles.

Obese people need to burn more fat and carbohydrates and may exercise gradually until reaching a set end goal. Exercise needs to be accompanied by a low calorie diet.

A person that consumes 2500 calories a day and is 20 pounds over their ideal or desirable weight needs to spend 2700 calories a day to achieve their goal in 3 months. Or else, spend 2500 and consume 2300 calories every day.

Exercise should not be viewed only as an activity aimed to improve physical health, endurance and provide muscle strength; rather, it needs to be appreciated in a larger context. In our culture it has a unique place in that it allows for social interaction, acceptance and a sense of belonging to a community of achievers and motivated people, since it also improves self esteem, helps fight depression and stress and provides an important sense of enjoyment and accomplishment.

Physical education classes in school or in other places have common aims, independent of which sport activity the student practices; the common denominator is that it builds discipline, an ethos, a e*sprit de corps*, a passion for performing, and a positive and optimistic attitude.

These features may get lost when we grow older and become immersed in other tasks but may be recovered by practicing recreational sports or physical activities with others.

5

When should we start practicing sports or gymnastics or physical activities and when should we stop?

Being sedentary has a damaging effect on our body and mind, so it follows that we should practice enhanced physical activity as often as we can, independent of age. Living a sedentary lifestyle has dreadful health consequences. Morbidity of all types is frequent. Obesity, cardiovascular disease, pulmonary infections, depressed immune system and inability to fight infections are among many of the ills associated with sitting and getting little exercise. Inactivity by choice or by design (as in the case of those who are deskbound because of their job) is injurious.

Children should start with programmed physical activities at age 3. It has been shown that regular physical activity helps in maintaining coordination and agility.

It is never too late to start. Alicia Alonso, who in December 2011 turned 91, is a famous ballerina and current Director of the Ballet Nacional de Cuba, who danced well into her late sixties and remains active.

In contrast, Marlon Brando, the cinematic icon who in 1953, when he was 27 years old, was seen in *A Street Car Named Desire* as a vigorous, strong young man, ended his life at age

80 weighing 300 pounds with diabetes, pulmonary insufficiency and cardiac disease; in the last three decades of his life he deteriorated physically and intellectually as a result of eating and drinking too much.

Independent of age, all exercise and strenuous physical activity should be done under medical supervision. A recent article published in *The Journal of the American Geriatric Society* showed that strenuous exercise in elderly persons is associated with an increased incidence of venous thrombosis. In contrast, a recent review article by Robert F. Zoeller in the *American Journal of Lifestyle Medicine* reached the following conclusions:

> The prevalence of overweight and obesity is increasing at an epidemic rate due physical inactivity.
>
> Increased adiposity, especially central or visceral adiposity, is predictive of cardiovascular disease, metabolic syndrome and diabetes, mediated probably by increased systemic inflammation, also as a result of being sedentary.
>
> Greater physical activity and/or fitness may reduce inflammation associated with greater visceral adiposity (in other words too much fat, too much swelling).
>
> Adiposity and low levels of activity and/or fitness are risk factors for atherosclerotic disease and Type 2 Diabetes, as well as the increased mortality associated with them.
> Increased physical activity/fitness reduces disease and mortality risk, regardless of Body Mass Index, but does not completely abrogate the risks associated with obesity.
>
> Both moderate to vigorous physical activity and weight loss independently reduce the risk of diabetes and improve glucose/insulin metabolism via different mechanisms.

Physical activity on the order of 2500 to 2800 kcal/week may be necessary to prevent weight gain or maintain weight loss.

Strength training is recommended as an adjunct to regular aerobic exercise but not as the primary mode of exercise for weight loss.

Individuals are strongly encouraged to engage in regular physical activity because of the known health benefits, regardless of whether that activity results in weight loss.

6

Where can we exercise?

Exercise can be performed in a diversity of places depending on personal choice, geographic area and financial considerations. Walking outdoors during the winter may be difficult but still may be practiced in big enclosed public places. The gym is a dedicated place designed specifically for physical improvement and they are everywhere--in schools, colleges, factories and a multitude of recreational places. Sports associations are built around a specific activity like soccer, rugby, rowing, horse riding, cricket, and others. Today exercising is part of an educational curriculum starting in kindergarten and continuing through university level. Physical activity is so entrenched in the American culture that over the last decades health clubs has proliferated and can be found everywhere; some are free, sponsored by localities, and others charge reasonable prices. If money are not available, there are a lot of public institutions that offer free or accessible physical fitness programs like colleges, YMCAs, senior centers, ethnic associations, churches and government agencies. Gym equipment can be purchased at sensible prices and gives the option of practicing in the comfort of home or office. The outdoors are fun and free and are always a good place to practice sports.

How many days a week should one engage in exercising?

Physical activity should be part of a daily routine. **Programmed exercise should be practiced at least five times a week.** A busy schedule is no excuse to skip what is essential for your health. Procrastination is a non-reflexive behavior that ends up producing undesirable effects on the body and mind. Postponing essential actions in life creates anxiety, stress and guilt. It has variable effects: at work it makes a person less productive, in a social context it may ruin relationships, and when it relates to health issues it has severe consequences--in the short or long run, it makes people sick. Enhanced physical activity is not as difficult to adhere to as dieting. People who are engaged in either a diet or in a physical program are more motivated to do both. The emotional and the physical rewards of spending energy are immediate. The release of endorphins and perhaps other substances like serotonin, epinephrine, dopamine and anandamide have been proven in multiple well-conducted investigations to be released by the pituitary gland in response to exercise, good stress, and other activities and are responsible for a sense of wellbeing, similar the one that others can get with recreational drugs but without the ill or deadly effects. The amount of time to exercise varies depending on sex, age, physical condition and associated diseases. In general terms 30 minutes is the minimal time, although for some older people and others 30 minutes may be too long, in which case it can be replaced with periods of 5 to 10 minutes, 2 to 4 times a day.

What are the drawbacks of exercise?

Stories of athletes, runners, joggers and others exercising and experiencing sudden death, independent of their fitness status, are not that uncommon. According to the medical literature, it occurs with a frequency of 1 in 30,000 to 100,000. Some runners without previous known disease die or suffer unexpected health consequences during long distance marathons due to the dislodging of a plaque in the circulatory system, producing a blockage of a coronary artery, or by the sudden onset of a cardiac arrhythmia produced by the release of substances that decrease the perfusion of blood to the heart, disrupting its synchronized function. Under strenuous conditions, heat and humidity produce excessive sweating, and this may deplete the body of electrolytes (salts), which are essential to maintain bodily functions.

These rare occurrences suggest that is a good idea to be pre-screened before starting on a program of exercise, independent of the anticipated level of intensity. Walking is an everyday activity that may not require doctor's advice, yet walking at a brisk pace or uphill may put a heavy load on the lungs and heart for somebody without previous training.

The minimal risks associated with demanding physical efforts are no excuse for not exercising because sedentary life carries worse risks in terms of morbidity and mortality than judicious training.

There is a strong professional and lay consensus about the benefit, impact, and influence of enhanced physical activity on the health of the population. It is, alone or in conjunction with sound nutritional approach, the more significant way to prevent infirmities. We live in a society that tends to provide comfort and ease to our daily existence. We don't walk to the store; we take our car even for few blocks. In China bicycling is the main form of transportation, with dedicated lanes on the streets. This may explain why Chinese people are so fit. In France three or four story buildings may not have an elevator, so climbing up the stairs is for some a common form of exercise. Fifteen minutes going up the stairs burns 100 calories. In Rio de Janeiro, people living in the hills walk, fetching heavy loads.

 We have to get rid of our lazy habits. Walking, running, moving, exercising and practicing sports is simple, cheap and rewarding and an essential part of staying healthy and fit. It helps to fight depression and stress and improves sleep.

Chapter 6

The Stress Chapter

Coping

It is not stress that kills us; it is our reaction to it.- Hans Seyle

1

From an early time as a physician, I learned that patients expressed their dysfunctional emotions, their solitude and their anguish with somatic manifestations. Stress made some of them sick, others with serious sickness got worse, while others reawakened a dormant condition. Latent diabetes may become overt after a stressful situation; some may develop a sudden heart attack after an unexpected event such as the loss of a dear one and many may develop an organic condition after a traumatic event. It is clear that a disease is more than an external agent deranging the human body and that there are other causes that make us sick, keep us sick or help us in getting well. Some with advanced atherosclerosis had no physical manifestations while others with milder forms had multiple complaints reflecting components other than a purely organic cause.

A surprising fact is that none of this was taught to medical students in medical school, not then and not now. The social, psychological and behavioral factors are part of the disease. Diabetes should no longer be defined as elevated blood sugar, but rather a condition that affects patients in certain way based on their own circumstances and where hyperglycemia is just one of its components. This explains why some individuals have a better or a worse presentation or a different response to exactly the same medication.

The advances in medical technology during my lifetime have been phenomenal. When I first started my practice, imaging of different parts of the body was rudimentary and inefficient. Later there was substantial progress in diagnostic and therapeutic equipment but the effectiveness did not translate fully into betterment of people's health. The ills of civilization increased at the same time that medical technology was achieving its best success. People in developing countries were afflicted mainly with conditions related to unsanitary conditions but as they evolved, they started suffering the same ailments that affect us. This happened when they began adopting our eating habits and polluting their environment like us. Leaving out smoking, alcoholism, drug addiction, crime and poverty, which are strong contributors to the decline of health, stress and insalubrious eating habits, lack of exercise and a contaminated environment are the most important elements in precluding our wellbeing.

Knowing the facts that interfere with the possibility of achieving perfect health (as perfect as their genetic makeup allows) is a first step. Pasteur once said, "Fortune favors the prepared mind." Knowledge is our responsibility and is the instrument to become truthful to ourselves and do something about it.

Stress is a constant strain in our health. Conquering stress facilitates staying fit and vigorous.

Recognizing problems is simple, but solving the paradigms is not.

Others and I, professionals and nonprofessionals alike, are advocating a return to simple habits. And yet we may be failing because our voices are being silenced by cultural leanings prevailing over reason and logic.

In previous chapters we have seen how the food industry is maiming us with insalubrious food, how the *comfort* of being bound to the couch watching TV, driving instead of walking and the pleasure of idleness are precluding our wellbeing and as we will see, stress adds to all these detriments.

We get stress (the third leg of health, nutrition and fitness being the two others) from the demands that society places on us, trying to keep up with the Jones, aspiring to get things we don't need, switching emphasis from spirituality to materialism, maiming our body and soul by internal and external factors and other events that shake down our emotional life and end up making us sick. We are enticed to consume beyond our needs. Recently, untidy consumerism, promoted by banks and corporations produced havoc in people's finances, creating all sorts of personal and social chaos. Many incurred debt above their means by utilizing their credit cards; others became unable to pay their mortgage or exhausted their savings that were earmarked to send their kids to college. Unemployment reached 12.4 percent. It is not difficult to imagine the associated stress from all those circumstances. The strength to cope with pressure, resolve conflict or avoid hassle is not easy to achieve. The result of a taxing life, a demanding routine or a hectic, nerve-racking existence is an angst that can either help us grow and become a better person or make us sick.

An epidemic of suicides in Greece and Spain in 2012 was the result of the stress caused by the financial crisis that affected more than 25 percent of their population.

When coping mechanisms fail, people may progress from transient benign conditions to more serious ones like cancer.

Stress develops when events become overwhelming and unmanageable. Occasional stress is part of everyday life and the way we manage it shapes our personality.

Relationships, getting married or divorced, problems with our kids, aging parents, financial crisis, retirement, and loss of capacity to earn needed wages, personal losses and fighting internal demons – to simplify a complex subject - may elicit a stressful response.

If the stressor is persistent and unmanageable, the individual may develop emotional symptoms readily recognizable as such, or they may masquerade as physical complaints denoting an unconscious defense mechanism.

Rage, fear, inability to concentrate, chronic fatigue, insomnia, anxiety and depression are some of the overt manifestations of stress, while tiredness, weakness, body pains and other physical ailments may develop when stress become unmanageable.

In 1965 I and others performed an investigation at Mount Sinai Hospital (today Cedars Sinai Medical Center) in Los Angeles, published later in the *British Medical Journal*, in patients with inflammatory bowel disease (IBD), namely Ulcerative Colitis and Crohn's Disease (which at that time were considered psychosomatic diseases), trying to determine if the cause was psychological in origin and also learn if these patients would develop a flare-up when they were under significant stress. The control group consisted of patients affected with other infirmities not considered to be psychosomatic in origin.

We found that IBD was not psychological in origin but that patients developed a significant flare-up after a stressful situation. To our surprise, the control group was also made sick by stress, which made us conclude that **emotional strain sparks off symptoms in all kinds of medical conditions**, independent of the primary cause.

Stress generates different responses in different individuals. Some start drinking or having an affair, or acting out, among other actions. In Argentina in the early 80s there was a severe financial crisis that affected the middle class and among other things, resulted in a significant increase in the divorce rate. This was interpreted as an acting out to relieve the emotional misery produced by their loss of status and money.

Traumatic events that are beyond our control, like rape, injury and assault, may cause what is known as a Post Traumatic Stress Disorder (PTSD), which manifests with extreme symptoms like insomnia, nightmares, inability to concentrate, uncontrolled anxiety and depression and other symptoms. Patients with PTSD may unconsciously recreate the original trauma, which perpetuates their symptoms, while many overcome the original injury and become stronger. Case in point: Mauricio Macri, the current city mayor in Buenos Aires, was kidnapped in 1991 and kept isolated in very confined conditions for two weeks, enduring a severe emotional trauma from which he slowly recovered; today he is fully functional, successful, remarried and aspires to become president of Argentina.

In 2008 Dr. Tarani Chandola and collaborators published an article in the *European Heart Journal* showing a definitive association between coronary heart disease and stress at work. They studied a cohort of 10,308 male and female civil servants based in London during a 12 year period. Those affected by stress showed decreased physical activity, poor dietary habits, unhealthy practices like smoking, and obesity. This association was stronger among employees younger than 50. The risk of myocardial infarction (MI) in permanently stressed individuals was associated with over twice the odds of MI compared with those reporting no stress at work.

In another study published in the *British Medical Journal*, the same authors showed that there was a positive correlation between stress at work and Metabolic Syndrome (MS). MS is used to describe a commonly found constellation of metabolic derangements that includes insulin resistance, hypertension, dislipidemia, and central or visceral obesity associated with accelerated vascular disease.

There is a large amount of scientific data that has proved without doubt the link between stress and organic disease.

2

The Libby Zion case brought workplace conditions in hospital settings to national attention because it was affecting medical residents' behavior, stress levels and patients' safety. Libby was 18 years old when she arrived in the Emergency Room at New York Hospital-Cornell Medical Center in New York the evening of October 4, 1984. The next day she was dead. On admission to the ER she presented with agitation, tremors and high temperature. She had a history of depression. Her family physician, Dr. Raymond Sherman, ordered her admission to the hospital ward. She was seen by a medical intern and a resident, who made a preliminary diagnosis of viral syndrome. She was agitated and according to the notes in the chart exhibited hysterical behavior. She was given Demerol, a pain medication that also produces sedation. Since she continued to be agitated, Dr. Luise Weinstein, the intern, was informed by the nurses of patient's condition and ordered restraint of the patient and an injection of haloperidol, a drug which is known to control agitated and aggressive behavior. Libby fell asleep. In the early morning her temperature was 107 degrees. Cooling measures were ordered, but Libby had a cardiac arrest and died. Her father looked into the situation and noticed that her daughter had been on Nardil, a monoaminooxidase inhibitor that precludes the use of Demerol because it enhances the strength and toxicity of the former. To make things worse, Dr. Weinstein was very busy taking care of other patients and Dr. Stone, the resident and first in command, was sleeping in his room during the incident since he had a very busy day. The case went to court, where it was made clear that doctors in training work under stressful conditions and are burned out and deprived of sleep, creating an environment where bad things can happen. This case underscores that working under stressful conditions is one of the factors responsible for the one million medical errors made every year in the US alone.

In the same area of concern, a study by Stucky and collaborators published in *Academic Medicine* showed in a group of 185 physician's trainees that work-related stress and poor sleep affected them and the safety of patients. Fatigue and stress were recognized as culprits. As a result, mandatory duty restrictions are now imposed in most medical institutions limiting working hours to 60 hours a week and limiting the on call duties.

3

The physiological and pathophysiological mechanisms of stress are being unveiled by multiple studies and provide the substratum to explain disease and behavior, giving an opportunity to manage stress by different means, including pharmacological intervention.

George P. Chrousos explains in *Nature Reviews Endocrinology* the mechanisms of stress and stress disorders:

Stress occurs when homeostasis is threatened or perceived to be so and homeostasis is re-established by various physiological and behavioral adaptive responses. The stress response is mediated by the stress system, partly located in the central nervous system and partly in different peripheral organs. The effectors of this system include the hypothalamic hormones arginine, vasopressin, corticotropin-releasing hormone and pro-opiomelanocortin-derived peptides and in the autonomic norepinephrine center in the brainstem and in the locus ceruleus. Targets of these effectors include the executive and/or cognitive, reward and fear systems, the wake-sleep centers of the brain, the growth, reproductive and thyroid hormone axes and the gastrointestinal, cardio respiratory, metabolic and immune systems. Optimal basal activity and responsiveness of the stress system is essential for a sense of well-being, successful performance of tasks, and appropriate social interactions. By contrast, excessive or inadequate basal activity and responsiveness of this system might impair development, growth and body composition, and lead to a host of behavioral and somatic pathological conditions. Our lifestyles and environment in modern societies seem to be particularly permissive for such stress-related disorders.

In simpler terms: constant strains, tensions and permanent hassles are responsible for initiating a cascade of biological events that impair mind and body and where almost every organ in the body becomes affected. When the response to stress is adequate, we return to a sense of wellbeing and no physical harm ensues, but when there is a failure to cope multiple body injuries can occur, some temporary and others permanent.

These basic concepts untangle the malfunction of our body when subject to a physical or emotional aggressor. Survival means to keep the house in order. We may allow a mild temporary disruption but repetitive offenses end up producing some dislocation in our psyche and in our body. There are conflicting reports regarding the association of stress and cancer; some investigations have indicated that chronic stress may compromise the immune system and trigger virus-associated tumors such as lymphoma. What is uncontroversial is that once a patient has cancer, additional stress may negatively affect the growth and spread of the tumor. This has practical applications because studies have shown that women with cancer of the breast have increased survival when participating in support groups aimed at decreasing stress.

Today we know that patients with Psoriasis, Irritable Bowel Syndrome, Coronary Artery Disease, Hypertension and other conditions get worse when they are under psychological stress.

The understanding of the link between mental and physical behavior and biology is providing a broader perspective of disease and allowing modification in management to prevent flare ups or recurrences.

Tuberculosis is produced by the Koch bacilli, yet not everybody exposed to it contracts the disease. Those who are resistant are protected by a balanced homeostatic mechanism, which includes a stable physical and mental state.

This puts infirmities in a more complete context, explaining why an external insalubrious agent may or may not affect an individual, depending on his organic equilibrium. Environmental, social, physical, mental and emotional factors contribute to this imbalance.

Managing stress, in addition to eating well and enhancing physical activity, is the mainstay for health support.

4

When I was Chief of Staff at Huntington Hospital I used to counsel some doctors who were under stress from malpractice litigation. One of them told me that he was afraid that he was going to lose his home although he carried enough malpractice insurance to offset all costs of litigation and compensation. He could not shake this impression; for him, being brought to litigation meant that he was a bad and an inefficient doctor with poor skills. That was his mental construct: 'I am no good; ergo I deserve what is coming to me.' I brought him to reality: he was as good as his peers, and he had a bad outcome in a particular case, which was not totally unexpected. A simple discussion was enough for him to be able to relax and cope. He settled the case. He confessed later to me that in order to protect himself, he is practicing "defensive medicine," which is bad for him and for patients, for him because he is not practicing to the best of his knowledge and for his patients because they are subjected to unnecessary tests.

Dealing with stress is part of the process of growth, a means to learn how to live our lives, confront tragedy and despair and in the meanwhile become more mature. The skills we acquire in confronting stress surely transfer to other spheres: work, family and social relationships.

One physician treated a young patient that had a vascular malformation (an abnormal conglomerate of vessels) in the stomach. He confused this lesion with a polyp, took a biopsy (which is absolutely contraindicated in somebody with this type of lesion) and the patient died as a consequence of unstoppable bleeding. The doctor became so distressed that he abandoned the practice of medicine. This is unfortunately one of the hazards of medicine, and physicians need to be prepared to deal with these kinds of situations.

About one million medical errors are committed in the US alone and as a consequence, about 100,000 patients die every year. Complications from medical or surgical intervention are not that uncommon and intrinsic to the practice of medicine; they produce stress to both affected individuals and physicians.

When somatic manifestations appear, it is important to visit a physician to assess if there is any organ dysfunction or failure that may need to be addressed immediately. **Stress can masquerade as an organic illness and organic illness can masquerade as psychosocial distress.**

In his book *How Doctors Think,* Dr. Jerome Groopman relates the case of a thirtyish year old patient who had seen many doctors over a period of fifteen years because of relentless lack of appetite, vomiting, nausea and abdominal pain. Since the subjective symptoms were apparently out of proportion to the objective findings, her physicians concluded that her symptoms were secondary to some emotional instability and sent her to see a psychiatrist, who made a diagnosis of anorexia nervosa with bulimia, a severe crippling condition that may be lethal. She was referred to several specialists, including psychiatrists and psychologists, and received multiple medications including antidepressants but to no avail. She developed anemia and had a bone marrow biopsy that revealed diminished cell production, which was attributed to severe nutritional deficiency. She also had severe osteoporosis. She tried to eat as much as she could to overcome her nutritional deficiencies, but the more she ate the worse she got. As a final hope she saw Dr. Myron Falchuk, a clinical gastroenterologist, who took a different approach. He made the correct diagnosis, when others had failed, by listening attentively to the patient and putting together all the pieces of the puzzle. After conducting some tests he diagnosed Celiac Disease. This is a condition where the surface of the small intestine becomes atrophic, impairing the absorption of nutrients and causing severe malnourishment. It is caused by an abnormal immune response to gluten, especially gliadin, present in certain foods, that when ingested produces damage to the mucosa within hours of exposure. The strict exclusion of gluten from the diet generally produces dramatic improvement and final reversal of symptoms. This case underscores the importance of placing stress in the right context. **Doctor Falchuk listened to the patient as a whole** and understood that patient's stress was caused by an organic condition and not the other way around, gave her some simple tests, made the right diagnosis, treated the patient with a gluten-free diet, and a result she got back to a normal state.

Porphyria is another condition that is many times misdiagnosed as a stress disorder because it has numerous symptoms, from abdominal pain, vomiting and constipation to back, limb and sensory loss. This diversity of symptoms makes diagnosis difficult and since patients' complaints are out of proportion to physical findings, patients are commonly diagnosed with a psychological disorder. This condition is an inherited or acquired disturbance of heme biosynthesis (the component that combines with globin to form hemoglobin) with overproduction and accumulation of porphyrin (a metabolic ancestor of the hem).

In our gastroenterology practice we have seen many patients with Celiac Disease and Porphyria who are usually referred with the wrong diagnosis of intractable Irritable Bowel Syndrome, the ultimate expression of a psychosomatic disorder.

Two other cases illustrate this quandary:

William R. was a 59 year old male who got over the grief from the death of his wife after nine months. He was enjoying life again, was productive at work and established a relationship with the widow of a friend. Two years later he started feeling depressed and somewhat tired. His family doctor felt that he was still mourning his wife, explained to him that it was a normal emotion and gave him a prescription for Zoloft, a common antidepressant. He then started having mild abdominal pain and lack of appetite; a CAT scan of the abdomen revealed a cancer in the body of the pancreas. It was his cancer making him depressed and not the purported grief over his wife's death; this underlines the fact that one may have had a stressful situation and then develop an unrelated organic condition.

The second case was of a 50 year old physician who I saw for evaluation of liquid diarrhea producing dehydration and electrolyte depletion. His condition was such that it required restoring the losses with frequent intravenous fluids. He was first seen by four different physicians, but no definitive diagnosis was made. The patient was in the middle of a divorce and this prompted all his doctors to assume that the diarrhea was secondary to stress. He was then referred to Dr. Isaac Lucchina, a famous psychoanalyst in Buenos Aires, who reached the conclusion that although the patient had some unpleasant life situations, overall he was coping well, was emotionally stable, was enjoying life with his children and did not exhibit any signs of stress. Lucchina became suspicious that something organic was going on, hence his referral. I performed a rigid sigmoidoscopy (the flexible scopes were not yet invented) that showed a villous adenoma very low in the rectum in an area of difficult access. Patient had the tumor removed surgically and all his symptoms disappeared. Although villous adenomas are not infrequent, this form of presentation is rather unusual. In most of the cases they secrete water and electrolytes which are reabsorbed by the colon, thus in that sense they do not produce ill effects, but when they are located very low in the rectum, reabsorption is overwhelmed and intractable diarrhea with the associated water loss ensues. This case gives emphasis to the need to differentiate emotional from physical disorders in order to reach the right diagnosis. In this case an astute psychoanalyst placed the patient in the right context.

I mentioned four organic conditions, which along with many others can impersonate as a functional disorder. Labeling a patient as having a stress-related disorder may be risky, the same way that not considering stress as the culprit of certain somatic manifestations is.

Not infrequently physicians don't take into account that physical symptoms may be related to stress and as a consequence patients get multiple tests and medications, when what is needed is to spend time patient to unveil some underlying stressful situation.

5

There are different approaches to managing stress. If one can recognize the cause--for instance, the loss of a job-- and cannot cope with the situation, one can get help from counselors, share the concerns with others or plan strategies to move on. Simple measures may reverse a negative circumstance into a positive one by setting goals and tactics.

Denial gives temporary comfort but long lasting pain. The anxiety generated by stress if not verbalized, internalized and clearly understood results in either behavioral problems or somatic complaints.

We talk more about stress reduction than stress elimination because we have come to terms that pressure, strain, worries, tension, hassles and traumas are part of our daily life. The first step in fighting the condition is to recognize the stressor and reflect about the cause and its consequences. Anxiety, frustration, rage and other symptoms after a physical or emotional incident may be transient phenomena but if they linger beyond a reasonable time, it is time to act.

A discussion of how a situation is affecting an individual and how he/she is handling it may help as a first instance. Sometimes it is easy to identify the stressor, while sometimes one cannot pinpoint a reason; for instance, when a co-worker is fired, it is not infrequent for others to fear that they are going to be next, even if there is no real cause to substantiate the supposition. When one experiences emotional discomfort and cannot pinpoint the cause, it is a good idea to take time out in order to identify possible stressors. This needs to be followed by an honest evaluation of the skills that one has to change or eliminate the offensive factor.

If simple measures like meditation, analysis, and sharing concerns with others do not mitigate or make the angst disappear, it is time to apply more advanced methods like relaxation techniques, breathing exercises, and imagery, techniques that should be learned from professionals.

When somebody is in a dire situation, an open discussion with friends or family or professionals is better than concealing facts. Planning a strategy to deal with a frightful event is the first step in resolving a crisis.

Chronic and unmanageable is stress requires psychotherapy and/or pharmacological intervention.

When the sun burns it is the right thing to look for shade and then be prepared for the next blaze. Running away from the glow requires too much energy and effort, both of which can be put to better use by building a place of safety; when the mind shelters our emotions by understanding our feelings we can move forward and shake off undue stress. Recognizing the essence of discomfort, acceptance and action are the best ways to deal with stress. Romancing what is worthwhile in life and throwing out the window what is not is the first step toward achieving emotional balance

Chapter 7

Promises and Betrayal

The Medication Chapter

Medications help, medications kill

1

In the early sixties during my gastroenterology (GE) training, most of our patients in the clinic were suffering from "heartburn," "indigestion" or "acid stomach," as we used to call the symptoms that today are known to be produced by gastroesophageal reflux (GERD). At that time we did not have fiber optic endoscopes, only rigid or semirigid instruments that were so brutal that we only used them as a last diagnostic resource. Our understanding at that time was that those patients had excessive hydrochloric acid in the stomach, causing gastritis (an inflammation of the lining of the stomach), and were treated with antacids. Patients usually responded to this kind of treatment and **we wrongly assumed that the hyperacidity theory was the correct one.** We learned decades later that in reality these patients had gastroesophageal reflux, a condition in which a normal amount of acid bathes the esophageal mucosa, producing an irritation at that level.

Our GE group was at the vanguard of research in Argentina. The chief of the Department at the National Institute of Health was Marcelo Royer, a world–renowned gastroenterologist who made important contributions in his field. He performed several studies in patients not responding to conventional treatment for their heartburn by performing a gastric analysis test, which consisted of removing acid from the stomach with a nasogastric tube. To our surprise, almost all of them had normal amounts of acid during basal state. The following step was to stimulate acid production with a meal or stimulants like histamine or pentagastrin to assess if eating was producing an inordinate amount of acid. Most of the patients with symptoms of "acid stomach" had normal values. This concept is so entrenched in our culture that today we keep miscalling reflux as 'too much acid' or 'acid stomach.'

Those patients who did not respond to the four times a day dose of liquid antacid, which was the standard recommended dose, had the amount increased to eight times a day, usually with good results. In other words, patients were treated for an assumed condition that they did not have, which luckily many times responded well to the simple, although cumbersome, frequent administration of an antacid.

The same treatment was given to patients with gastroduodenal ulcers. Most of them responded well but there was a small subset that required major surgery, not exempt of morbidity and mortality.

At that time the frequent administration of antacids was considered a scientific truth, although we were wrong in the tenets of acid stomach, gastritis and peptic ulcer disease; nevertheless, we were doing the right thing with the only available treatment to protect the lining of the upper gastrointestinal tract.

Then things changed:

In the sixties the fiberoptic upper endoscope was introduced by Dr. Basil Hirshowitz, first with the use of an endocamera, which consisted of taking an inordinate amount of pictures of the stomach and analyzing them one by one. Later an optical system was developed which allowed viewing the stomach directly and obtaining biopsies. This revolutionized the field of gastroenterology, which changed to a more precise discipline.

GERD was redefined and explained. Heartburn, acid stomach, indigestion, and dyspepsia were produced by the normal acid of the stomach in contact with the lower esophageal mucosa when the sphincter (ring) between these two organs became incompetent. This is called Gastroesophageal Reflux (GERD). The therapeutic principle, though, was the same: cut the production of acid as much as possible.

We learned a lot about function and dysfunction of the stomach, but treatment continued to be unsatisfactory. Antacids, gels, and Reglan (a medication to move the acid away from the esophagus) were used with some success, while other patients remained sick.

In 1976 a new medication transformed the way we treated GERD and ulcers. The discovery that there were two histamine receptors H1 and H2 in the stomach, and that by blocking the latter gastric acid could be diminished, led to the discovery of cimetidine (Tagamet) which was followed by the development of ranitidine (Zantac). These classes of medications are called H2 antagonists. They became the first medications to surpass the billion dollar mark in annual sales. They were effective; the side effects were minimal and manageable; and they were helpful in controlling GERD and stomach and duodenal ulcers. For us as gastroenterologists, they represented the second revolution in our field, the first being the introduction of endoscopy.

Years later the third revolution occurred. A new medication, omeprazole (Prilosec), was launched. At the beginning they called it Losec, but pharmacists, because of doctors' famously poor writing, used to confuse the name with Lasix, a water pill, thus the name change. This was also an acid suppressant medication but acted by a different mechanism than H2 blockers. They inhibit the pump responsible for initiating acid formation so they are known as proton pump inhibitors. They were exceedingly effective compared with H2 blockers.

Prilosec became one of the best-selling medications in the world and rightly so. It was, in our and in our patients' minds, a miracle medication. It was effective, had few side effects and was safe and easy to take. GERD patients were no longer awakening in the middle of the night with burning or regurgitation. Used in conjunction with lifestyle modifications like reducing weight, avoiding foods that are known to decrease the lower esophageal pressure and sleeping with the head of the bed elevated, Prilosec made symptoms disappear. GERD, a onetime unbearable and distressing condition, became easy to manage.

At that time, there were other impressive achievements in the field of pharmacology:

Oral hypoglycemic agents were developed, allowing millions of patients to stop injecting insulin.

Chemotherapeutic agents were expanded and reversed the fatal outcome of many cancers.

The introduction of these medications and many others represents the best of pharmaceutical companies. Developing medications takes effort, creativity, perseverance, patience and money. The development of a drug needs to be followed by strict clinical trials to assure that it is safe and that the benefits outweigh potential harm beyond any doubt. The task of R&D is monumental and has greatly benefitted humanity. It was, is and will be responsible for extending life and providing comfort and wellbeing to billions.

The list of accomplishments of the pharmaceutical companies is long and impressive. Unmistakably, they deserve the gratitude of society, but...

2

The push to use medications curtails the possibility of alternative ways of treating disease. As an example that can be extended to the majority of medications, the proton pump inhibitors (PPI)--Prilosec, which they called the purple pill, (now an over-the-counter med), Nexium, Axid, Zegarid, Kapidex, Prevacid, Aciphex--are being advertised extensively and used indiscriminately. They are usually safe but not exempt of side effects or undesirable interactions with other medications such as coumadin, digoxin, iron supplements, antifungal, Plavix and some antiretroviral medications. GERD should always be managed with a concomitant lifestyle modification, which should include weight reduction; avoiding foodstuffs that are known to decrease the lower esophageal sphincter (the ring that separates the esophagus from the stomach), such as chocolate, mint and fatty foods; smoke cessation and sleeping with the head of the bed elevated. After achieving control of symptoms PPIs should be stopped. But since it is easier to take a pill that change our ways, drug companies take advantage of this by bombarding patients with their ads and TV commercials to increase consumption. **This is a significant problem because as a consequence there are millions of people taking this medication when they could do without it and be served much better by modifying poor habits.**

When the patent for Prilosec was about to expire and become generic, Astra Zeneca, the manufacturer, introduced a new PPI, Nexium, which was achieved by slightly modifying the chemical structure of Prilosec. All of a sudden Prilosec became a second rate medication. Nexium was aimed to replace it because it was 'able to confer better protection, heal esophagitis faster and avoid response variability.' What they never mentioned is that the variability was minimal. Prilosec, once it became generic, cost 14 dollars versus $172 for a month's supply of Nexium. Nexium suddenly became the 'purple pill'. Is Nexium better than Prilosec and better than other generic or non-generic similar drugs? Ask any gastroenterologist and most of them will tell you that they are all very good and that the response variability can be resolved by increasing the dose or switching from one generic to another. It is clear that there is no reason to prescribe costly drugs when similar, less costly alternatives are available.

How Astra Zeneca did persuade doctors to prescribe Nexium? What you are about to learn applies to a multitude of other drugs and reflects the practice of almost every other drug manufacturer.

This is my personal experience: In the eighties, all of a sudden, by the grace of a Pharmaceutical Company I became a gastrointestinal consultant. The representative for the company invited me to share my "expert opinion about a new medication." I was flown from Los Angeles to New York, lodged in a first class hotel and given a 1000 dollar honorarium. The next day I attended a meeting where other invited gastroenterologists were present to discuss PPIs and hear about a new one. We were divided into small groups and a discussion leader commanded the discussion. The meeting was animated, the gathering cordial, and we all went back home convinced that there was now a promising new drug in our armamentarium. Alas, it took more than a year for me and others to realize that we had been duped. That meeting was the way to introduce a new PPI to physicians. In this instance I was neither an expert nor a consultant but a tool in their marketing designs.

Prilosec and Nexium are similar; the latter marginally better in investigation trials but not in everyday practice. This is one of the many ways that drug companies may impose a new medication with a huge potential for sales and which in realty is no better than its predecessors.

Other ways of enticing the use of "name brand" medications, in lieu of cheaper versions, is to offer them at a discount price to hospitals or managed care organizations, although always more expensive than the generic counterpart. Pharmaceutical companies treat doctors lavishly, first with all kinds of gifts, and now that this practice has been prohibited by the government with new schemes, like organizing dinners in fancy restaurants to discuss medical related topics, discussions that last no longer than few minutes as not to impact the doctor's leisure time.

The practice of introducing similar drugs with similar therapeutic benefits is the way that pharmaceutical companies have to increase their pockets at the expense of the consumers. Marcia Angell in her book *The Truth about the Drug Companies* calls them Me-Too drugs, meaning a new version of an old one, an effort that is financially rewarding because it cost little to develop a variation of an old one. By placing them in the category of a new drug they get a new patent which is good for 20 years. These new meds don't have to show that they are better than their counterparts, only that they are better than placebos; the implication is that they may be worse than existing drugs.

Clarinex replaced Claritin; they are practically identical. Statins, antidepressants and others that generate high sales belong to the family of Me-Too drugs.

Pharmaceutical companies entice the consumption of medications by advertising them directly to the consumers. As a result we have become a nation of pill takers, and physicians a cadre of pill pushers.

Greed from drug companies is tainting their important contributions, because medications can cure but they can also kill.

3

The cholesterol dilemma:

The first statin was lovastatin, which was isolated from a fungus. Since then there has been an explosion of similar drugs, each claiming to be better than the other. Millions of persons are taking statins to reduce their cholesterol and others with normal cholesterol also take them to decrease the risk of coronary artery disease (CAD), the rationale being that it diminishes plaque formation, thus preventing myocardial infarction. A load of research appears to demonstrate that statins may also prevent stroke and peripheral vascular disease and **perhaps** cancer of the colon and prostate, hypertension, cataracts and lung cancer.

The competition among pharmaceutical companies in general is enormous and more so with statins since they generate billions of dollars in yearly revenue. The financial reward is so big that today seven companies in the market are battling each other for the largest piece of the pie. The chemistry of statins is very similar, as are their therapeutic benefits so in order to have an advantage over each other pharmaceutical companies resort to different gimmicks to increase their market penetration, including aggressive and creative promotion, conducting clinical studies with the hope to show some comparative benefit and aggressive advertisement to physicians and to patients. The patent of some had expired and now simvastatin (generic for Zocor) is selling for four dollars a month, competing with atorvastatin (Lipitor), which sells for about 150 dollars. One would expect that both being similar, simvastatin might outgrow Lipitor in sales, but that is not the case, mainly due to aggressive advertisement for the latter. Another trick to increase sales is to combine them with another medication; Advicor is a combination of a statin with niacin that lowers LDL; Caduet contains a statin and a calcium channel blocker to decrease blood pressure.

It is expected that 36 million people will be taking statins in the US alone, which is more than ten percent of the population. There is ongoing joke about statins claiming that they are so effective that they should be added to drinking water.

In 1997 Bayer jumped on board with Cerivastatin (Baycol), asserting superiority in comparison with others. Marketing and sales were brisk, but in 2001 they withdrew the drug from the market because it produced several deaths attributable to rhabdomyolysis (destruction of skeletal muscle tissue), which led to renal failure. Some of these patients were also taking another anticholesterol drug, Gemfibrozil, and it appeared that the combination of both was more harmful than each one alone. A medical review concluded that this medication was 16 to 80 times more likely than other statins to produce a breakdown of skeletal muscle cells with its nefarious consequences. Bayer was sued by many patients and settled for 477 million dollars, a dent to a company that has annual sales of 48 billion dollars. An article published in 2003 in the *New York Times* stated that senior executives were aware of the serious and undesirable side effects of the drug long before they pulled it from the market. This was revealed in sworn depositions, e-mails and memos and they acted only when they had no other option.

The story of statins does not start or end here since there are many questions related to safety, taking a medication for life, side effects and alternative ways of lowering cholesterol. **The subject is important and confusing.**

High cholesterol is not a medical entity in itself, the same way that high blood sugar, high potassium and low sodium are not. Coronary artery disease, diabetes, kidney disease and dehydration are the conditions where those kinds of abnormalities are present. The distinction is important because, for example, hyperglycemia can be treated with a low carbohydrate diet and lifestyle modification while diabetes is a well defined disease that requires constant and aggressive therapeutic intervention. The same concept applies to cholesterol.

Before we can make treatment directives with certainty, based on science we need to answer the following questions:

* *Of 100 patients with high concentration of cholesterol, how many will have a heart attack or a stroke?*

   Answer: A study of 100 patients showed that the risk is about 3%.

* *Lipitor manufacturers claim that "... in a large clinical study, 3% of patients taking a sugar pill or placebo had a heart attack compared to 2% of patients taking Lipitor." This in practical terms means that for every 100 patients who took the pill over 3.3 years, three on the placebo and*

two on Lipitor had a heart attack; the sensible question then becomes: is it worth the risk of side effects and cost for the other 97 people to take the pill?

Answer: The crucial dilemma is how to identify that extra patient who may benefit from a statin to avoid treating a large population in order to save one life. What we should be doing is improving outcomes by decreasing cholesterol level by other means since it is known that **lifestyle modification decreases the incidence of coronary artery disease better than statins alone, as revealed by coronary angiograms according to a study that showed regression of lesions of 10.7 for lifestyle versus 2.1 for statins, an impressive finding.**

- *Of 100 patients with high concentration of cholesterol due to high HDL (the good one) and normal or low LDL (the bad one), how many are in danger of developing a heart or brain problem, thus needing to take anticholesterol meds?*

    Answer: Since HDL is protective, most likely there is no need to treat patients with normal or high HDL, even if the total cholesterol is high. High cholesterol should not be treated without measuring LDL (although since LDL constitutes 60 to 70% of total cholesterol, in the absence of LDL measurement one may assume that it may be high). Nowadays, it is inexcusable not to get a complete lipid profile before treatment. If LDL is above 160 mg/dl and the patient is high risk for CAD (for instance with a strong family history of cardiac ailments, or a previous heart attack, or being morbidly obese), drug therapy should be considered; if the patient is no or low risk for CAD and the LDL is below 189 mg/dl dietary treatment is in order and if this does not correct the problem consideration of drug therapy should be entertained.

- *Is low cholesterol bad for your health?*

Answer: Low cholesterol is usually a manifestation of liver failure, thyroid disease and other associated ailments. If it is produced by drug therapy, the dose should be corrected or the medication suspended.

• *How is a high level of cholesterol defined?*

Answer: Cholesterol above 200mg/dl is 'abnormal', but if the HDL accounts for most of this amount and the LDL is normal, the total cholesterol figure becomes irrelevant. An example: Total Cholesterol: 220 mg/dl, HDL 100 and LDL 120.

• *What is the effect of lifestyle modification (diet, exercise, reducing stress, smoke cessation) alone in reducing cholesterol and how does it compare with drugs alone?*

Answer: This is a crucial question. Multiple studies have shown that drugs are better than diet alone in decreasing the incidence of heart attacks (not necessarily degree of CAD), 24 vs. 30 percent, and mortality, 21 vs. 29 percent. But note that diet is still an effective treatment. And further: on those studies no other lifestyle modifications (like smoke and alcohol cessation, stress reduction, etc.) were applied that may have offered a better outcome. A sensible, yet not proven assumption is that removing all high risk factors and a proper diet may be as effective as or better than drugs alone.

• *What is the role of triglycerides?*

Answer: Triglycerides are a definitive risk factor for CAD and can be lowered by lifestyle modification--to be more specific, by **weight reduction, increasing physical activity, smoke cessation, stress reduction, low carbohydrate diet, limiting alcohol and controlling associated conditions like diabetes and certain drugs like corticosteroids and estrogens**

• *What is the optimal therapeutic approach to prevent a heart attack?*

Answer: This is the state of science today:

Hypertension should be vigorously treated. Although it does not remove the risk 100 percent, it contributes significantly in lowering its incidence. Cigarette smoking should be absolutely prohibited. Associated conditions like diabetes should be treated. Obesity is a major modifiable factor, as is physical inactivity. Atherogenic diets (containing trans fats, polysaturated acids and high carbohydrate content) increase LDL and should be discouraged.

- *Are there better markers or indicators of heart disease than cholesterol?*

  Answer: There are multiple serum markers that may able to define who is at risk for a heart condition or who should be treated but they are not applied in clinical practice, either because they are expensive or difficult to measure, like apolipoproteins, lipoprotein remnants, small LDL particles, lipoprotein a, HDL subspecies and others. There are also non-lipid risk factors like homocysteine (very likely), atherogenic factors like platelet aggregation (thus the therapeutic effect of aspirin, which prevents this phenomenon) and inflammatory markers like C-reactive protein, impaired fasting glucose, coronary calcium and the metabolic syndrome. Seldom are those parameters taken into consideration, and this omission precludes identifying the population that is truly at risk.

- *Is there a cause for high cholesterol and would we be better off if we target the cause?*

  Answer: Cholesterol may be increased by excessive consumption of fats but in certain individuals it is due to a metabolic abnormality that is not well understood.

- *Since many of the cholesterol guidelines have been developed by professionals that had received or are receiving money from drug companies, how trustworthy are their recommendations?*

Answer: These professionals make their conclusions about statins suspicious at best; consciously or unconsciously receiving money from drug companies may be a factor in emphasizing their virtues and minimizing their defects.

- *Are there better drugs than statins to increase the good cholesterol?*

    Answer: Nicotinic acid has been shown to effectively increase HDL. This medication carries less significant side effects than statins.

From the above discussion it is clear that:

We don't have all the answers about who may benefit with absolute certainty from statins, with the exception of those with high risk factors.

There are millions who are taking these medications needlessly*. This is due to poor understanding of the totality of the cholesterol paradigm by physicians and by patients, by the lack of adherence to lifestyle modification measures, by ignoring the effect on cholesterol of associated morbid conditions, by eating the wrong stuff, by not incorporating plant stanols/sterols like soybean, commercial margarines (providing to adjust intake to account for the calories they provide), and tall pine tree oils, by not eating enough viscous fiber-containing edibles like oatmeal, psyllium, beans and pectin-rich fruit and by decreasing animal fat intake.*

Other alternatives include nicotinic acid or lipid sequestering medications and, as we mentioned, removing modifiable risk factors like diet, smoking and excessive weight and controlling associated morbid conditions

Family history of coronary artery disease is a clear indication to take statins, but only when the above other strategies have failed.

Omega 3 fatty acids present in fish or in capsule form, canola oil and vegetable oils in general, English walnuts and soybeans are definitive ways to prevent heart events such as myocardial infarction and sudden death.

Folate and antioxidants should be consumed daily and mainly in the form of edibles and not drugs. Supplemental vitamins like vitamin E, beta carotene or others may not be needed. **Dietary sources of antioxidants are better sources than supplements.**

Moderate intake of alcohol may be beneficial in lowering the risk for coronary events, while large amounts have the opposite effect.

Soluble fiber, cereal grains, fruits, vegetables, dry beans, legumes and plant stanols/sterols (present in special margarines, soy proteins) are beneficial. Losing weight lowers LDL, as does enhanced physical activity. Folate from dietary sources may decrease the incidence of CAD. The Institute of Medicine recommends a daily dose of 400 mg, not to exceed 1000 mg. Herbal or botanical dietary supplements are not recommended since they have not shown any meaningful benefit and furthermore may interfere with other medications. Sodium intake should be less than 2,400 mg/day. Magnesium, calcium and potassium are part of a healthy diet. Drug therapy should be considered a last resource.

In summary:

High cholesterol, when it is due to increased LDL, is an independent high risk factor for Coronary Artery Disease, but it should not be contemplated in isolation. It is important to consider the affected individual as a totality: weight, dietary habits, smoking, alcohol, stress, abdominal girth, stress, life situations, family history, associated morbid conditions, education, gender, ethnicity, family or peer support, among many other factors. All these factors should be pondered to better outline a treatment plan, which should consist mainly of lifestyle changes and the use of medications as a last

<u>resort</u>. Against this is the culture of medication popping, fomented by pharmaceutical companies, through pandering to physicians and other tricks of the trade. Two extraordinary books on this subject are *Selling Sickness: How the World's Biggest Pharmaceutical companies are Turning Us All into Patients* by Ray Moynihan and Alan Cassels (Nation Books,2005) and *The Truth about the Drug Companies: How they deceive and what to do about it* by Marcia Angell, ex-editor-in-chief of the New England Journal of Medicine (Random House, 2004). Those books are very revealing in their discussions of the way the pharmaceutical industry operates. It exposes their devious practices, the influence they have in lobbying Congress to achieve their designs, the eschewed relationship with the Food and Drug Administration, their entanglements, marketing practices and mainly the damage, that is, injury and/or death. One of the more damaging actions is blasting consumers with advertising, so detrimental that no other country in the world, with exception of New Zealand, allows such a practice. If I ask the reader to pay attention to pharmaceutical practices, it is because it is a train that may, contrary to popular belief, be taking you to a destiny of despair.

Other factors that contribute to the abuse of anticholesterol medications are careless physicians for whom it is easier to write a prescription than to devote time to learn about his/her patient's life situation and to spend time with them to counsel for the best available treatment option and by the health care delivery system that puts more emphasis on treating people than preventing disease. And finally by those of us who don't assume the responsibility to do what is right for our health.

4

Novartis voluntarily withdrew Zelnorm, a medication used for Irritable Bowel Syndrome, because of excess risk for angina, heart attacks and stroke, rectal bleeding and abdominal pain. This was the responsible thing to do but what was not responsible was the unrelenting advertisement of the product in the media to increase consumption prior to removing the medication from the shelves.

In 1985 the FDA approved Seldane, the first prescription antihistamine to relieve allergies without causing drowsiness, a great advance compared to others, which, while relieving symptoms, were making patients sleepy. A few years later the medication was discontinued because it was found it could cause fatal cardiac arrhythmias when used concomitantly with drugs that slowed their elimination from the body, or in patients with liver disease, but not until after aggressive direct-to-consumer ads that made the manufacturer billions of dollars.

Vioxx was a new class of antiarthitic medication successfully introduced in 1999, with annual sales in the billions of dollars, but it was withdrawn from the market in September 2004 because of a fourfold increase in the risk of myocardial infarction. Several patients or family members on their behalf brought litigation to Merck, the manufacturer, who by now has paid almost one billion dollars in compensation. The essence of the dispute between Merck and the plaintiff's lawyers was the issue of malicious intent by their top executives to defraud the public. Merck itself conducted their own investigation that showed that although they acted honestly, an overzealous sales team exaggerated the safety of the drug and withheld valuable information about its perils. The *New England Journal of Medicine* entered into a dispute with the authors of a published article about the supposedly beneficial effects of the drug, accusing them of withholding information about its pernicious effects.

Cipro, a widely used and advertised antibiotic, was given to postal workers as a preventive measure after alleged anthrax attack. A class action suit was later brought against Bayer AG because of unexpected side effects that included tendonitis, tendon rupture, anxiety and depression.

I recently visited a friend of mine who had a cast on his foot. He underwent an uneventful cholecystectomy for acute cholecystitis. Upon discharge he was given Levaquin, a medication similar to Cipro. After few days he experienced severe pain on his left foot caused by a rupture of the Achilles tendon a known complication of this kind of drugs. It took him almost one year of treatment and rehabilitation to get well. He was never told by the prescribing physician or the pharmacist of this dreaded side effect. This case underscores the potential problems that this, as so many other medications, may cause.

Several other medications have come and gone after being on the market for years when the ill effects outweighed the benefits. In almost every case the pharmaceutical companies have been brought to trial. Drug companies have been accused of not posting warning labels to alert patients of undesirable or fatal consequences, downplaying their side effects or hiding their pernicious actions.

Zyprexa (bipolar and schizophrenia), Serzone (depression), Prempro (menopause), Rezulin (diabetes), Paxil (depression), Fosamax (osteoporosis), Meridia (obesity), and Ketek (antibiotic) have serious side effects, are still on the market and have all been litigated in court. To be sure, some of these, if carefully prescribed by physicians, are useful and effective, but only a professional can balance the pros and cons of all medications. **Advertising influences patients who demand prescriptions from their physicians and taints their decision making.**

Phen-pen (weight loss), Bextra (antiarthitic), Celebrex (antiarthitic), Redux (obesity), Propulsid (dyspepsia), and Ephedra (herbal stimulant) have been banned and are no longer available but not before they were consumed by millions and maimed or killed many patients.

There are 1.3 million pharmaceutical errors committed every year from the 3 billion prescriptions written in the US alone, producing from minor to fatal injuries, a problem compounded by an unrestricted consumption produced by the lure of commercial advertisement.

The FDA is the federal regulatory agency that has the obligation to ensure that drugs and medical devices are safe and effective and yet many times after drugs have been approved they are discontinued because of injury and death beyond reasonable expectations.

Many medications are legally used off-label by physicians, a practice that in some cases produces more harm than good.

Medications need to be taken only when needed, used cautiously and discontinued when the therapeutic target is achieved. These premises are seriously undermined by pharmaceutical companies, which takes us to the next story...

5

Mr. X is afflicted with cancer and undergoing chemotherapy. He feels tired and is leery that he won't be able to work in the bed and breakfast hostel he runs with his wife. He decides to ask his doctor about Procrit, which he prescribed. Next scene: Mr. X feels much better and is shown working again in a scene where he is greeting his guests.

Mr. Y, an auctioneer, is on chemo and for the first time in 30 years he feels so tired that he is afraid that he might not be able to work in a subsequent antique auction. Next scene: He asked his doctor about Procrit and after getting the drug feels well enough to go back to work.

 "**Procrit** is safe; only diarrhea and edema may occur..." The voiceover announces.

These are two of the many commercials that were run on national television advertising Procrit (known as ESA, or erythropoiesis-stimulating agent), a medication that when applied correctly is very effective. This drug stimulates the bone marrow to produce red cells and is used to correct certain types of anemia without transfusions; it is administered when the red cell count reaches critically low levels and only in conditions that cannot be treated in other ways. Procrit has been misused in patients with transient anemia from chemotherapy. It has been given in many cases as a quick fix with fatal consequences, as in some patients with chronic renal failure (who characteristically are afflicted with anemia), who have experienced greater risks for death and cardiovascular events such as myocardial infarction, stroke, congestive heart failure, and vascular access thrombosis when on hemodialysis. These undesirable effects have been reported in a randomized, prospective trial of 265 hemodyalisis patients.

Another well controlled study with another ESA (Epoetin alfa), performed in 939 women with metastatic breast cancer receiving chemotherapy performed to study survival rates compared to placebo, was terminated prematurely when interim results demonstrated a higher mortality at four months (8.7% vs. 3.4% for placebo) and a higher rate of fatal thrombotic events in the first four months of the study. Also, an increased incidence of deep vein thrombosis (DVT) in patients receiving Epoetin alfa and undergoing surgical orthopedic procedures has been observed. In addition, increased mortality was observed in a randomized placebo-controlled study of Procrit in adult patients who were undergoing coronary bypass surgery (7 patients in 126 patients randomized to Procrit versus no deaths among 56 patients receiving placebo).

Some patients with advanced head and neck cancer receiving radiation treatment, others receiving chemotherapy for metastatic breast cancer or lymphoid malignancy and others with non-small cell lung and other malignancies receiving chemotherapy or radiotherapy had increased mortality and/or increased risk of tumor progression or recurrence after being treated with ESA medications.

Decreased overall survival was observed in four other clinical studies and decreased progression-free survival and overall survival was documented in three other investigations.

In another study, red cell aplasia (inability of the marrow to produce red cells), a fatal hematological disorder has been reported, which is the medication producing the opposite of what is intended to do. Another undesirable side effect from this medication was the appearance of seizures in patients with chronic renal failure (CRF).

ESAs have been a definitive advance in the medical field and have definite advantages. Many patients with chronic renal failure have been able to improve their hemoglobin levels on their own, obviating the need for frequent transfusions. Patients with HIV infections and certain cancers also have benefited from this class of medications but Direct-to Consumer Advertising (DTCA) of medications promoted unnecessary consumption.

In summary, Procrit, which at one time have been heavily advertised in the media as a safe and effective drug, is not free of significant side effects and it has produced unexpected fatalities. Advertisement of this medication on TV has now stopped but not until after it increased consumption, leading to injury and death, by its aggressive marketing.

DTCA creates a dangerous culture of drug consumerism, as much as street drugs do. Since the legalization of DTCA, the use of prescription medication increased by more than 30 percent. This is a subject that has not been addressed by physicians or by the government and as a result, we are in a quagmire. More medications mean more opportunity for side effects and increased cost of care. Money spent on advertisement of medications would be better spent on health education and prevention.

The *Wall Street Journal* reported that doctors who attended a dinner conference sponsored by the manufacturer of Vioxx wrote nearly four times more prescriptions than their counterparts. This medication, as we mentioned, was withdrawn from the market because of its serious side effects.

Pharmaceutical companies claim that public advertisement of medications is a form of making patients aware of their existence and consequently benefitting from them. This is a nonsensical subterfuge. Advertising medications boosts sales by the billions, while in the process some may get hurt, injured for life, crippled or die. We are prone to believe the written word and images when they serve our illusions.

The problem is compounded by the fact that physicians are easy prey and part of the problem. Marketing is a formidable weapon that penetrates the minds of physicians and dictates their actions. We are dined and wined, given gifts, invited to exotic places and paid fees as 'consultants' as a way of enticing us to prescribe their products. For many professionals the cornucopia of attention is difficult resist. Most of us honestly believe in our own incorruptibility, without realizing how subliminal advertisement, gifts and other gimmicks can affect our prescription habits.

Drug companies not only use perks like gifts, invitations to concerts and sports events and free samples but also employ concealed approaches like hiring reps who are young and attractive and know how to engage doctors in selling their products. Carl Elliot wrote a piece called *The Drug Pushers* in *The Atlantic Monthly* in April 2006 and posed a provocative question: are doctors becoming the new drug reps? It was unsettling to read that reps call some of these doctors "drug whores."

James Reidy, a drug sales representative for Pfizer, Inc. and Eli Lilly and Co. who was fired after writing a book about his experiences, said that "drug companies seduced doctors with escalating financial inducements that often start with paid trips to learn about a drug."

Dr. Richard Grimm of the Berman Center for outcomes and clinical research in Minneapolis, who himself earned more than $798,000 from drug companies in an eight year period, said

"Drug companies are like lions. For lions, it's their nature to kill zebras and eat them. For drug companies, it is their nature to make money. They're not really trying to improve anybody's health except if it makes them money" (*New York Times,* 03/21/2007).

The efforts by the AMA and government agencies to avoid the unwanted influences of the drug companies resulted in new regulations, which have been easily circumvented by new marketing strategies.

6

According to a major clinical study by the Antihypertensive and Lipid Lowering Treatment to Prevent Heart Attack Trial (ALLHAT), hypertension should be treated first with lifestyle modification and the use of generic thiazyde diuretics. This first line of action is not applied by physicians as often as it should be, depriving patients of the chance to use less expensive and safer treatment modalities.

The ALLHAT trial revealed the merits of a medication that costs 13 cents a day versus Norvasc, a calcium channel blocker that costs $2.73 a day.

The recommendations of this panel were soon ignored because the makers of patented medications responded to the results of this trial by redoubling their marketing efforts and trying to discredit the results of the studies.

Comparative effectiveness studies are essential to elicit the best therapeutic alternative. This is how the ALLHAT trial came about. They compared a diuretic (chlorthalidone); an ACE inhibitor (lisinopril); a calcium channel blocker (amlodipine) and an alpha blocker (doxazocin). What was learned was dramatic: the cheap diuretic was better as a fundamental line of treatment and furthermore, doxazocin, an expensive antihypertensive medication, was dropped from the study because it caused significant heart failure.

ALLHAT, which was organized by the federal government, could save billions of dollars since there are millions of patients with hypertension taking the less qualified medications, but this is not happening because of the pervasive and insidious efforts of the drug manufacturers influencing physician practices.

Later, a new study, ACCOMPLISH, showed that the best combination is that of an ACE and a calcium channel blocker, but the dose of the diuretic (chlorthalidone) given in that investigation trial was not optimal.

I am discussing this complex situation for the reader to understand that there is chaos in the treatment of hypertension, and this calls for caution.

Educational measures, enforcing standards, demanding strict adherence to protocols, peer review, and health organization intervention are potential ways of making sure that patients get the best available and not the best marketed product, but this is not happening.

Fewer medications means fewer side effects, drug dependence, and expenditure and switching from a drug culture to one of self reliance.

7

Medicalization of habitual life situations is one of the more dangerous artificial creeds created by drug makers. Grief caused by the loss of a loved one has been transformed into a depressive condition requiring antidepressant medication; occasional disinterest in sex because an individual may have other things in his mind, like difficulties in his job, financial problems, bad relationships or whatever has been labeled as sexual impotence necessitating Viagra; sexual difficulties by women led to a new syndrome, Female Sexual Dysfunction (FSD), a situation that can be 'cured with a testosterone patch', which is now a 1 billion dollar market.

All these inventions ignore the complexity of life circumstances, where not only biological but psychological, situational, cultural, environmental and existential factors play a role. Aging manifestations like osteoporosis, diminished stamina, wrinkles, fat belly, blood pressure, cholesterol levels, sleeping difficulties, decreased libido and others have been medicalized to the extent that now they are considered medical entities and, like other medical entities, are treated with medication, ignoring better alternatives like, for example in the case of osteoporosis, exercising and a diet rich in vitamin D and calcium and sun exposure. Insomnia managed by sleeping pills instead of stress reduction is an example of the overuse of drugs. There is a new class of medications to treat insomnia, like Ambien, Lunesta and others which should be used only for very short periods of time, such as when traveling or preoccupied by recent concerns; unfortunately, there are many using these drugs on a regular basis, not taking into consideration the harmful side effects like behavioral changes, abnormal thinking, and sleep driving, to name only few of the reported collateral problems.

Bayer is targeting the weariness that most of us experience when we wake up in the morning by aggressively advertising Bayer AM, an over-the-counter pill that contains aspirin and caffeine. Aspirin can cause gastrointestinal bleeding among other side effects and caffeine can cause cardiac arrhythmias. To be more emphatic: medications can help, medications can kill.

Inventing new diseases brings a huge, profitable market to pharmaceutical companies; the disregard of concerns about safety and benefits is appalling. It creates a civilization of legal drug takers, which is as bad as the one of illegal drug consumers.

In most instances what is needed is lifestyle modification.

8

Robert Boyle, who lived in the seventeenth century, is considered the father of chemistry. He had an analytical mind and made efforts to understand the nature and composition of matter. He was an alchemist, preoccupied as others at that time in transmuting or converting metals into gold. Herbal medicine and modern medicine came about at the same time, when chemistry and physics were nascent and evolving and utilizing the same principles of alchemy. Belladonna is the quintessential herb, literally and figuratively speaking; it contains an active substance that now has been synthesized in the lab and converted into the active ingredient of many medications. It contains alkaloids like atropine, scopolamine and hyoscyamine and has remedial and cosmetic effects. The synthesis of Belladonna (which translated literally means beautiful woman, from the fact that the plant was used to dilate their pupils, conferring a luscious and attractive demeanor) is an example of alchemy at it best.

Ephedra is a plant that contains ephedrine and pseudoephedrine, both of which have extensive use in medicine. It was first used in China 5000 years ago. Opium, aspirin and digitalis have also their origins in plants.

These and others have enriched our modern pharmacopeia. Twenty-five percent of today's medications are derived from plants, and this explains why in many cultures herbalism is still the predominant form of therapy.

When orthodox medical practice is ineffectual, some patients resort to non- conventional treatments.

In primitive societies treatments were administered by tribal healers using plants as an adjuvant to their magical powers. The 'empacho' is a folk illness of children characterized by unrelenting colicky abdominal pain, at times associated with nausea and vomiting. Some of us, with strict scientific positions, have seen pediatricians advising parents to call a 'curandero' (a witch doctor of sorts) when they could not help a kid get rid of the problem. The curandero would pull the wall of the abdomen while at the same time chanting a prayer to their indigenous gods, resolving in minutes what appeared to be an otherwise unmanageable problem, underscoring that there are still a lot of things we physicians don't know.

Herbal medicine, a discipline practiced by honest licensed physicians, groups and institutions, is also a terrain populated by charlatans or unscrupulous persons. There are very few herbal remedies that have been shown by rigorous scientific clinical trials to be effective in humans and animal experiments.

Herbal manufacturers sell billion of dollars of plant remedies in dedicated stores, supermarkets and pharmacies; they don't need approval by any regulatory agency providing that they label them as nutritional and not therapeutic. There are more than 50,000 herbs being sold in the US. Herbs don't undergo the rigorous testing required for prescription drugs. *Consumers Reports* magazine in the 1010 September issue reported 12 herbal products that the Natural Medicines Comprehensive Database deemed unsafe. They are Aconite, Bitter Orange, Chaparral, Colloidal Silver, Coltsfoot, Comfrey, Country Mallow, Germanium, Greater Cellandine, Kava and Yohimbe, producing all kinds of significant ailments including heart, kidney, liver and brain damage. Deaths have been reported in patients taking Bitter Orange, Lobelia, Aconite and Yohimbe.

Herbs create an illusion of wellness, which explains their 'beneficial' effects. Some manufacturers of herbal supplements added drugs like steroids, sildenafil (Viagra) or appetite suppressants intentionally to enhance the effectiveness of inactive herbs, a clearly illegal practice that can be dangerous and even lethal.

This brings us to a crucial question: do herbs have any place as a therapeutic alternative to conventional treatments? The answer is a qualified yes. Fish oil, lactase, psyllium, and probably cranberry, lactobacillus, Pygeum and SAMe and others have shown a definitive value in preventing (not treating) certain conditions, while more than 95 percent of others have never proved to be as effective as they claim and are not exempt from side effects.

Taking multivitamins is a routine practiced by millions, generating a multibillion business, a habit difficult to explain since we can satisfy all our vitamin needs by a comprehensive diet, which in addition provides required fiber and phytochemicals such as the ones contained in fruits and vegetables. Only those with nutritional deficiencies, restricted diets, chronic disease conditions and pregnant or breast feeding women benefit from vitamin supplementation.

Medications and herbs deserve scrutiny to prevent harming those they want to help. The FDA is the institution responsible for approving and running the checks and balances on prescription medications, but time and again they fail to do so, as illustrated by not the infrequent recall of some of them.

Fosamax (alendronate sodium) is a widely used medication for the treatment of osteoporosis. This medication can cause from minor to debilitating adverse reactions and most of the time the problem is resolved by discontinuing the medication. In a few instances irreversible severe osteonecrosis of the jaw and fracture of the femur can occur. This led to class action litigation against Novartis, the drug manufacturer. The occasional yet sometimes very serious side effects explains the reluctance of some people to take this or other medications and seek alternative treatments that may not carry unwanted risks. Pigweed leaves, garlic tablets, parsley, and dandelion are been offered, without demonstrable validation, as an effective treatment to halt or reverse osteoporosis. Therefore women who are commonly affected with this condition usually face a therapeutic dilemma that needs to be addressed by a physician with an ample comprehension of the problem because not all the cases are the same and should not be treated with a cookie-cutter prescription.

Individual herbal species are being tested in randomized clinical trials in well established, respectable medical institutions. This is being performed because there has been a clamor by the population to find alternative means of treatment with plants with no undesirable side reactions and low cost, and without the need to visit a medical doctor. For the moment these are unfulfilled promises. A careful reading of the findings from the National Center for Complementary and Alternative Medicine (NCCAM), a federal government agency for scientific research practices and products, created in 1992, will convince the reader that there are very few herbal supplements that deserve to be part of their medicine cabinet.

Let's take for example Cat's Claw (Uñas de gato), an herb that grows in the Amazon rainforest that has been used for centuries to treat disease and today is advocated as a cure for Alzheimer's, cancer, HIV, preventing or aborting pregnancy, supporting the immune system, promoting kidney health and preventing arthritis. The conclusion by the NCCAM is that none of the claims are valid. How do we then explain its popularity? The Amazon symbolizes nature and provides the oxygen we breathe and is a habitat uncontaminated by civilization, therefore we assume that whatever originates there should be pure, useful and safe, and we get carried away by promises that are almost invariably false.

Another popular herb is St. John's Wort, which has been used for centuries to treat mental disorders and depression, usually administered as teas prepared from its flowering tops or as tablets containing concentrated extracts. In spite of its widespread popularity, the herb was not more effective than a placebo in treating major depression, according to a study sponsored by the NCCAM.

Multiple herbal trials are currently being conducted in patients with nausea secondary to chemotherapy, patients with

Ulcerative Colitis, others with degenerative diseases and palliation of terminal patients, so far with negative results.

Memorial Sloan Kettering Cancer Center is conducting quality of life studies using botanical elements, to further advance this subject.

Garlic is recommended by herbalists as a potent anticancer herb, or to treat high blood pressure or osteoarthritis, but these claims have never been supported by scientific evidence.

Milk thistle, advertised to help liver function, AIDS and cancer patients, has been shown to be ineffective.

One of the most popular and best selling natural remedies is glucosamine-chondroitin and MSM preparations.

A large-scale, multicenter clinical trial in five different groups was performed in the US to test the effects of glucosamine-chondroitin used separately or in combination in reducing pain in patients with osteoarthritis. The study, called GAIT, was conducted in 16 rheumatology centers across the US and coordinated by the University of Utah School of Medicine. For comparison participants received also celecoxib, a known proven antiarthritic med and a placebo. Researchers found in 1,583 patients with osteoarthritis that:

Participants taking the celecoxib experienced statistically significant pain relief versus placebo. Overall, there were no significant differences between glucosamine and placebo with the exception of a subset of participants with moderate-to-severe pain where glucosamine combined with chondroitin sulfate provided statistically significant pain relief compared with placebo; about 79 percent had a 20 percent or greater reduction in pain versus 54 percent for placebo. According to the researchers, because of the small size of this subgroup, these findings should be considered preliminary and need to be confirmed in further studies.

For participants in the mild pain subset, glucosamine and chondroitin sulfate together or alone did not provide significant pain relief.

In follow-up studies assessing the x-rays, data showed no improvement in slowing the loss of cartilage in osteoarthritis of the knee in a study from the Mayo Clinic staff, confirmed in 2009 by researchers at the University of Pittsburgh.

In summary there is no strong clinical evidence about the benefits of this widespread herb. Interestingly, the studies showed that patients with osteoarthritis respond positively to placebo in more than 50% of the cases, which highlights the power of the mind. (Source: NIH)

The current limitation of natural products should not preclude the investigation and assessment of the value of herbs and other complementary forms of therapy. Not too long ago probiotics were dismissed as ineffectual. Today they are making a comeback since preliminary studies have shown them to help patients with irritable bowel syndrome, diverticulitis and inflammatory bowel disease.

9

Antioxidants are substances that protect the cells from the damage caused by free radicals (unstable molecules made by the process of oxidation during normal metabolism). Free radicals may play a role in cancer, heart disease, stroke and other diseases of aging. Antioxidants can be found in edibles that contain beta-carotene, lycopene, vitamins A, C and E and other manufactured elements.

Several laboratory studies have shown that antioxidants may slow or prevent cancer, although some randomized clinical trials reached inconsistent conclusions. Some were positive, showing gastric cancer prevention in a Chinese Cancer Prevention Study in 1993 by using, beta-carotene, vitamin E and selenium, while two studies showed **increased** lung cancer rates with the use of Beta-Carotene and vitamin A.

There are multiple foods rich in antioxidants:

Beta-carotene is found in orange, sweet potatoes, carrots, cantaloupe, squash, apricots, pumpkin and mangos. Also in spinach and collard greens.

Lutein, associated with healthy eyes, is abundant in green, leafy vegetables.

Lycopene is a potent antioxidant found in tomatoes, watermelon, guava, papaya, apricots, pink grapefruit, and blood oranges.

Selenium is a mineral, not a nutrient. However, it is a component of antioxidant enzymes. Rice and wheat are the major dietary sources in some countries, while in the US meats and bread are common source. Brazil nuts contain large quantities of selenium.

Vitamin A is found in liver, sweet potatoes, carrots, milk, egg yolks and mozzarella cheese.

Vitamin E, also known as tocopherol, is found in almonds, in many oils including wheat germ, safflower, corn and soybean oils and is also found in mangos, nuts, broccoli and other foods.

Tobacco and radiation and exposure to other environmental factors can lead to free radical formation. In humans the most common of free radicals is oxygen. When an oxygen molecule becomes electrically charged or "radicalized," it tries to steal electrons from other molecules, causing damage to the DNA and other molecules. Over time, such damage may become irreversible and lead to disease, including cancer. Antioxidants are often described as "mopping up" free radicals, meaning they neutralize the electric charge and prevent the free radical from taking electrons from other molecules.

Studies are being performed to learn if green tea can prevent heart disease, dark chocolate can control hypertension and improve the response to insulin and if ginger and turmeric can reduce inflammation associated with arthritis and asthma.

In this context, foods in a symbolic way are medicinal, having significant protective and curative properties.

Antioxidants are also delivered in medicinal form, although it is always better to obtain them from fruits and vegetables because they also contain fiber and other beneficial ingredients.

10

In Summary:

We have grown dependent on prescription and nonprescription medications in the form of herbs or nutritional supplements. Effective medications usually carry significant side effects in contrast with the ineffective ones. There is no question that medications save millions of lives but unfortunately they also kill an estimated 200,000 people a year in the US alone. Some of these deaths are a consequence of unforeseen circumstances or when medications are given knowing potential risks, which are outweighed by the benefits. But in many cases medications are given without consideration to safety or potential side effects, or when they have not been tested long enough, mainly because regulation of the drug industry is lax and inadequate. The globalization of the pharmaceutical industry has created different venues for them to avoid scrutiny in our country. Conducting clinical trials in other countries makes it easy to present results that are spurious or blatantly false and as a consequence people have gotten sick or died.

There are new cadres of companies that perform medical trials for pharmaceutical companies to collect medical information, for example (and I have known this first-hand), to perform upper endoscopies to assess the effectiveness of an already established medication. For this, doctors are paid an honorarium per patient. In principle there is nothing wrong or unethical with this; patients are informed that they will be included in a research protocol and sign an informed consent and the medication is a known entity and the instrumentation is a well-established diagnostic tool. The problem is that very seldom do doctors know about the results of the trial, how exactly the data is being collected and analyzed and who exactly are the people responsible for the entire operation, and so doctors sometimes inadvertently become the pawns of a scheme to defraud the public.

Drug companies have as a priority to remain profitable and as a consequence have failed in providing safe and effective medications all the time, as they should.

The last medication that epitomizes the failing of pharmaceutical companies is Avandia. This is an antidiabetic medication that was presented to physicians and the public as one of the foremost advances in drug therapy. It effectively was able to control blood sugar elevation. Many years after its introduction (after becoming an extremely profitable medication, in the billions of dollars) the FDA estimated that Avandia had caused 83,000 heart attacks in an eight year period (and consequently many deaths); as a result of this the drug was banned in Europe, while in the US it is still in use, although Glaxo, the manufacturer, has stopped its promotion. In the meantime it has settled more than 11,000 lawsuits. It is disconcerting that having excellent alternatives for the treatment of diabetes, this medication is still available in pharmacies all over the US.

Direct –Consumer-Advertising is responsible for inducing people to consume an inordinate amount of medications which, besides creating a culture of pill pushers and pill poppers, have maimed and killed many.

Many of the readers may believe that the description of the ill-practices from drug manufacturers disclosed above may have been isolated incidents that I and others are depicting in order to advance an ideological agenda against the corporate world as an expression of opposition against free enterprise. This is far from the truth; on the contrary, an honest capitalistic society, incorruptible, which has the interest of people at heart and resists making a profit at all costs, is the ideal for a free society. Our country is the pioneer in technological advances, has created goods that have served humanity beyond anybody's imagination and need to continue to do so with trustworthy ways. To make my point about deceiving practices, I have excerpted an article published in the *New York Times* on October 27, 2010: *...GlaxoSmithKline, the British drug giant has agreed to pay $750 million to settle criminal and civil complaints that the company for years knowingly sold contaminated baby ointment and an ineffective antidepressant – the latest in a growing number of whistle-blower-lawsuits that drug makers have settled with multimillion dollar fines. Altogether, GlaxoSmithKline sold 20 drugs with questionable safety that were made in Puerto Rico that for years was rife with contamination...In a rising wave, recent lawsuits have asserted that drug makers misled patients and defrauded federal and state government that, through Medicare and Medicaid, pay for much of health care.* In the same article a graph shows that *...Pfizer paid a total of $2.3 billion dollars in fines for problems related to Bextra, Geodon, Zyvox, Lyrica and nine others; Eli Lilly $1.4 billion for Zyprexa violation, AstraZeneca $520 million for Seroquel, Bristol-Myers Squibb $515 million for Abilify...*among others (to be sure: this case refers to illegal marketing and in the case of GlaxoSmithKline to contaminated products).

Devious companies and unscrupulous individuals, under the pretext of free commerce and freedom of expression, sell insalubrious products, entice people to take medications that they don't need and create artificial or useless products that we consume or use, so they can get rich, all of which have a dire effect on us.

Herbal therapy seldom is effective, which calls for a serious discrimination of what is good and what is bad in the arena of alternative treatment modalities.

Chapter 8

Before The Storm – The Prevention Chapter

The prevention of disease today is one of the most important factors in the line of human endeavor.- Charles Mayo

1

The path of health is more than a balanced approach to a sensible lifestyle, eating well, exercising and reducing stress.

I know an individual who at age 56 had fairly normal eating habits, normal weight, played tennis once or twice a week and attended a gym on a regular basis. One Sunday, in the early morning while sleeping in bed he became restless and started panting. His wife thought that he was snoring hard, tried to wake him up but with no success. He was breathless. She tried an improvised CPR and called 911. In two minutes the San Marino, California paramedics were in the house. The gentleman was in full cardiac arrest, no pulse, no breathing. He was connected to a defibrillator, shocked once, and carried to the hospital three miles away. In the ER he was intubated, placed in a respirator and received IV fluids. A cardiologist, who had been alerted before the patient arrived, took him to the Cardiac Lab. An angiogram revealed a narrowing of the left main coronary artery, known as the widow maker, because frequently the obstruction kills the patient. The obstruction was relieved by angioplasty; the patient was transferred to the Coronary Care Unit, where he stayed for three days. His family was anxiously waiting for him to wake because the concern was that the lack of oxygen to the brain that he had during the cardiac arrest may have produced a cognitive or physical impairment. As is customary, while he was intubated he was kept under sedation and that precluded an early evaluation. Finally, on the fourth day he woke up with his mentation and motor functions completely intact. Family and friends could not believe that David, a symbol of health, had a heart attack.

I know this patient well. It was me.

After recovery I had a thorough evaluation. Prior to this I never visited an internist. I had occasionally checked my blood pressure in the office and it was occasionally mildly elevated. I had once some laboratory tests, including measurement of total cholesterol, which were within normal limits.

The cardiologist explained that I had a small myocardial infarction that precipitated the arrest. My blood pressure was mildly elevated, and although the total cholesterol was 168 milligrams, a surprisingly normal value, the Low Density Lipoprotein (which I never measured before) was high, consistent with a factor known to be responsible for plaque formation in the coronary arteries. Joel Heger, my cardiologist, asked me about my family history. I explained that my dad died at age 37 from a heart attack and his other 10 siblings had a strong history of heart disease. He looked at me and said nothing--he didn't have to--but I could read an admonition on his eyes. I was placed on hypertensive medication, baby aspirin and Simvastatin, an anticholesterol medication. I get periodic checkups once a year and have been well since.

Could my cardiac arrest have been prevented? The answer is yes. Any person with a strong family history of heart disease should have a cardiac evaluation consisting of a physical examination, an electrocardiogram, blood tests including a total lipid panel and a CRP (C-reactive protein) and a stress treadmill test, as a minimum. In my case it would have revealed an abnormal Low Density/ High Density Lipoprotein ratio and very likely the stress test would have shown signs of low perfusion to the heart at certain levels of physical effort. In other words, I could probably have prevented the cardiac arrest. It would have saved my family the aggravation, sorrow and despair that they went through and prevented my near-death experience. There are about 340,000 cases of cardiac arrest in the US yearly, and only 15 percent survive. These grim numbers emphasize the need to put prevention in the front burner, a notion that applies to this and multiple other diseases.

My omission could have cost me my life and caused my family devastation. In financial terms my stay in the hospital was very onerous. My health insurance paid, but the economic burden was shared by the rest of society.

This brings me to the core of this chapter. Very few people are actively engaged in an active, routine prevention program, an incredible situation. We responsibly maintain our car in driving condition, our house in a livable state and yet fail to adhere to a plan to stay strong and healthy.

We can prevent the mind and body from declining prematurely by undertaking preventive measures that cost little money but require a major personal effort.

2

Preventive Medicine is conveniently divided into: primary, secondary and tertiary.

Primary Prevention refers to **reducing** risk factors that can affect the integrity of the body and slow the inexorable aging process. Genetic makeup is a factor in determining the fate of our health but only to a certain extent. We cannot change our genes and yet we might be able to modify some of them for the better.

We need to follow simple steps. Simple means straightforward, yet at times difficult, demanding and strenuous but feasible and rewarding.

These are primary prevention steps:

- Eating the right amount of good quality food
- Maintaining an ideal weight
- Exercising daily – Aerobic and Resistance modalities
- Periodic medical check ups
- Taking medications or supplements only as needed
- Absolutely no drugs or smoking; alcohol only in moderation
- Avoiding pollutants
- Managing stress
- Not ignoring physical or emotional symptoms, as they may be the warning signs of an impending sickness

Those assertions are like the truths of Perogrullo, a fancy, chimerical character, an invention of somebody's imagination, perhaps the famous author Francisco de Quevedo, who expressed obvious truths in a simple manner such as: *"a closed hand is a fist," "when is hot is not cold"* and other trivial affirmations.

If anyone doubts of the consequences of living amiss, here they are:

Smoking, excessive alcohol and drugs are injurious and in the long run lethal and represent the most deleterious elements of our civilization.

Smoking kills every year about half a million people in the United States alone. Cancer of the lung, bladder and pancreas, peripheral vascular disease, coronary artery disease, laryngeal leukoplakia, chronic obstructive pulmonary disease, and cancer of the tongue are proven tobacco-induced conditions.

Alcohol in excess is responsible for the development of fatty liver, liver cirrhosis, pancreatitis, depression, panic disorders, neuropathy, gastritis, urinary incontinence, Wernicke's encephalopathy (characterized by confusion, loss of equilibrium and peripheral neuropathy) and dementia.

Drug addiction is secondary to a variety of agents, exerting its effect by stimulating the central nervous system, such as amphetamines, or by producing a hypnotic action, such as barbiturates, or sedatives and opioids producing analgesia and a sense of artificial wellbeing, such as morphine and codeine. Heart disease, psychiatric disorders, physical dependence, kidney failure, hemorrhagic or ischemic stroke, destruction of the nostril cartilage, suicidal ideation, lung disease are just some of the ill effects of drug addiction.

The health implications of all these addictions are enormous, while the social repercussions represent one of the most pressing issues of modern civilization. The description, analysis and treatment of addiction are beyond the scope of this book, but it suffices to say that there is no way of achieving good health without stopping the use of drugs.

Pollutants of any type produce different kinds of acute and chronic conditions. The most common occupational diseases that can be readily eliminated by avoiding exposure are: Asbestos is responsible for mesothelioma of the lungs or abdominal cavity, an inflexible, fatal condition. Carpal tunnel syndrome, a common condition affecting the median nerve of the hand, produces motor and sensorial changes at that level, affecting poultry workers and other occupations; byssinosis produces pulmonary disease due to the inhalation of cotton, flax and hemp dust and affects textile workers, and pneumoconiosis affects coal miners. The list of these poisons is large and the reader should be alert to their working conditions to avoid occupational hazards.

Complex and creative research has existed since Pasteur and Jenner initiated a cascade of measures that we use today in preventing disease. Pasteurization and vaccines were initial breakthroughs responsible for saving millions of lives, while today we can preempt the appearance of disease by multiple means.

Vaccination is a primary preventive measure that has positively influenced the disappearance or amelioration of disease. Tuberculosis and poliomyelitis are in part things of the past. Hepatitis B virus, diphtheria, tetanus, measles, mumps, rubella, pertussis, rubella, influenza, and pneumococcal pneumonia are the most common vaccinations that are effective when administered at the right time at the right dose in well-defined age groups. Travelers are recommended to be immunized with various vaccines depending in epidemiological factors of the countries to be visited, like cholera, plague, typhoid, yellow fever vaccines rabies, hepatitis A, Japanese B encephalitis, polio and meningococcal meningitis.

Vaccination is not without controversy. Some people refuse to vaccinate their children and themselves on religious grounds. Others are afraid of the side effects that may arise from immunization, while some claim that they trigger other unexpected conditions like autism, a most discussed and written about condition. It is not surprising that there is concern about vaccination, a method applied to healthy individuals that may end up harming them. Yet smallpox and polio have been almost completely eradicated thanks to vaccination. It is true that polio vaccine reportedly caused paralysis in a **very few** cases, which is to say that it provoked the condition that it wanted to prevent. On the other hand, the vaccine has been administered by the millions and millions avoided contracting the disease. The benefits of immunization outweigh the potential for harm by a long, long run. Autism was never proven to be caused by vaccination and yet is a big scare for many parents, and as a result some refuse to provide their kids with the most elemental and most needed immunization. Aluminum, which is used in vaccines in very small amounts to enhance their immunological potency, has been blamed without scientific validation as neurotoxic.

Some claim that compulsory vaccination curtails freedom of choice and avoid their use and yet doing so is a socially irresponsible action because a sick kid may infect others. The common good in society supersedes individual liberties, as is the case of not allowing driving a car on the wrong side of the road.

The swine flu is a universal epidemic that killed thousands of persons in 2010. An H1V1 vaccine was developed at incredible speed and was dispensed to millions of individuals. This prevented a calamity and yet some have taken a strong position against its use. One of the more vocal enemies of vaccination is Bill Maher, a brilliant political satirist with a large audience, who tweeted that those who get the vaccine are idiots. In other forums he tried to explain his position against some vaccines in-depth and he ended up making deeper nonsense. The World Health Organization has recommended immunizing high risk populations, including pregnant women, with the swine flu vaccine. It is unethical and inconceivable that public figures with access to millions of people are taking a wrong stand, without scientific basis, jeopardizing the health of others. It is true that people should not be taking every scientific claim at face value since again and again what appeared to be right today may be wrong tomorrow, but one has to live life accepting certain values. Today science is OK with vaccines and serious scientists are on the alert for adverse effects.

Hygienic habits, like practicing hand washing as frequently as needed, minimize the risk of contracting unwanted disease a practice that is encouraged especially among health workers, those who work in a kitchen and all others who interact with crowds.

The maintenance of optimal dental hygiene is important in preserving health. Many conditions affecting different organs have their port of entry in the mouth, which is full of bacteria that can turn deadly in special circumstances. For example, patients with certain heart valve conditions may develop inflammation of the lining of the heart, a serious condition, when undergoing teeth cleaning by a dental hygienist because instrumentation may dislodge bacteria from the mouth that may find their way into the heart, calling for these and other patients to take antibiotics before having some dental work.

Avoiding exposure to sunlight and using potent sunscreens is highly effective in preventing the appearance of melanoma, a dreadful disease that affects about 175,000 people yearly in the US and kills about two-thirds of them. Booth tanning, once considered safe, appears to produce or predispose to skin cancer as well.

Health prevention goes hand-in-hand with maintaining a good state of nutrition, sleeping well and managing your emotional wellbeing.

Accidents are among the leading causes of infirmities, together with cancer and heart disease.

Using seat belts while driving, wearing helmets when biking, workplace safety measures, not talking on the cell phone, text messaging or multitasking while driving, the implementation of anti-locks brake and air bags in automobiles, and environmental protection actions are all compulsory measures that have increased our safety net.

Government agencies, health professionals, schools, and the workplace are responsible for designing primary prevention measures and making sure that they alert and inform everybody about the perils of toxic products. Campaigns against smoking have effectively decreased smoke consumption and consequently led to a decrease in the incidence of cancer. In certain states dispensing soft drinks and snacks containing too much fat and calories has been prohibited in schools with the aim of decreasing childhood obesity, which is reaching calamitous proportions. Scientific societies are publicizing the importance of certain screening methods for cancer prevention, such as mammograms, colonoscopies, pap smears and other tests. All these efforts may be ineffective, however, if individuals don't take responsibility for their actions. A combined personal and societal commitment would make prevention a real accomplishment.

3

Secondary Prevention refers to **uncovering** disease before it strikes. There is a large group of medical conditions that can be diagnosed in their early stage and by doing so making them manageable or disappear altogether.

Doctors, physicists, geneticists, biologists, engineers and others have developed over the years an armamentarium to diagnose dormant or potential medical problems before symptoms arise. Others have strategized means to avert communicable diseases. As a result, we are today in the incredible position to arrest disease before it hits. This has tremendous individual and societal implications. Becoming a healthy nation would practically solve the cost of providing medical services overnight. This is not an exaggeration because it is accepted and recognized that most our infirmities are diseases of civilization. Genetics, casual pathogens, and other non recognized factors also play a role in initiating disease and sometimes there is little we can do to avoid them. But even those conditions can be reversed, halted or made better by early diagnosis and taking simple measures. Proper nutrition and weight control have been shown to reverse gene alterations that are part of the aging process, hoping that if the genes become younger, we may live longer. You will be reading more later about telomeres, the markers of youth.

This is a list of conditions that can either be detected before they appear or diagnosed during early stages, the connotation of which is that fate can be twisted:

Cancer of the colon
Cancer of the prostate
Cancer of the esophagus
Cancer of the uterine cervix
Cancer of the breast
Melanoma –other Skin cancers
Diabetes
Hypertension
Glaucoma
Tooth Disease
Oral cancer
Heart Disease
Infections
Stroke

Cancer of the Colon:

When President Ronald Reagan had surgery for a localized colon malignancy it led to an upsurge of diagnostic colonoscopies, soon to be forgotten. When Katie Couric's husband died at an early age of colon cancer, she almost single handed initiated a campaign for colon cancer prevention and even had a colonoscopy on live TV. This public campaign was incredibly effective in alerting people about the risks of contracting colon cancer and how to prevent it; and soon we gastroenterologists could not keep with the demand for colonoscopies.

This was understandable because the incidence of cancer of the colon is about 150,000 new cases a year in the US accounting for about 50,000 deaths.

Early detection involves, among other things, a simple fecal test for occult blood in the stool, independent of age. This is usually performed at the time of a physical examination and is performed by the doctor, who obtains a small amount of stool for a smear during a routine digital examination of the rectum.

People with a family history of colon cancer or polyps are considered high risk and advised to have early checkups and more thorough investigations.

Colon cancer almost always starts like a benign polyp formation, which means that its detection and removal prevents this lesion from transforming into a malignancy. Ninety percent of colon cancer occurs in individuals over the age of 50.

Colonoscopy is recommended in asymptomatic patients over the age of 50 at different intervals, depending on the findings, and earlier in those with familial adenomatous polyps, ulcerative colitis and Lynch syndrome (a form of hereditary nonpolyposis) and family history of colon cancer.

Cancer of the Prostate: About 230,000 patients will be diagnosed with cancer of the prostate every year and about 30,000 will die from it. Screening is performed by a digital examination that may reveal a nodular formation in the periphery of the gland and by measuring PSA (Prostate Specific Antigen) in the blood, which is elevated in 2/3 of patients with cancer, which means that another 1/3 may have the condition with normal values. Transrectal ultrasound and biopsies usually follow an elevated PSA. The management of prostate cancer is controversial because there are multiple treatment alternatives, from surgically removing the prostate to attacking the gland with different types of radiation or criotheraphy (freezing the gland) **or doing nothing** since cancer of the prostate may grow very slowly and an affected individual may die from other unrelated conditions. This last assertion has been corroborated by autopsy findings of cancer of the gland in patients who were completely asymptomatic and not known to be affected with the disease. In cases of metastasis, medical or surgical castration produces androgen deprivation that slows its progression.

Finasteride is a medication that blocks the conversion of testosterone to its active form and is used to treat benign prostatic enlargement (hyperplasia) and recently was found to decrease the incidence of cancer by 25%. There is no association between a large prostate and the appearance of cancer. The question being discussed at this writing is if prescribing Finasteride as a preventive measure makes sense or not. The medication is not exempt of side effects such as breast enlargement and decrease of sexual libido, which makes the decision rather difficult. It is always best to discuss prevention and management with a urologist because of the complexity of this entity. One should not rush to surgery because the operation carries risks and complications. Lately two reports claimed that statins, which are used to treat high cholesterol, may coincidentally decrease the incidence of cancer of the prostate, but it is too early to take this as an incontrovertible truth. Selenium and lycopene, which at one time were supposedly preventative, were shown to have no salutary effect. Supplements of folic acid in amounts larger than required and low fat milk with added vitamin A may trigger cancer of the prostate. This underscores the discussion about using nutritional or dietary supplements wisely.

Herbalists and those selling nutritional supplements to prevent or cure cancer of the prostate are providing false hopes and a disservice to affected individuals. Billions of dollars are spent every year in the consumption of useless pills. Saw palmetto, which has sold by the billions of dollars claiming to be the magic preventative pill, has not shown to prevent the onset of prostate cancer, according to a study published in the *NEJM* on February 9, 2006.

There are doubts among scientists that lycopene, which is a powerful antioxidant found mainly in tomatoes, can prevent this condition. Selenium, although proven to be protective in rodents, has failed thus far to prevent any type of cancer in humans. Beta-sitosterol, advocated for preventing and treating cancer of the prostate and breast, has never shown to do what it promises. The same is true for antioxidants like green tea, broccoli, cabbage and vitamin E.

Cancer of the Esophagus: Some patients with chronic gastroesophageal reflux (GERD) may develop a pre-cancerous condition called **Barrett's** esophagus, where the cells at the level of the lining of the distal esophageal mucosa start resembling the cells of the stomach. Over time the abnormal local mucosa may become dysplastic (a change in the morphology of the cells) that may progress to cancer. Treatment of GERD should be undertaken, although symptom control does not guarantee halting the progression from Barrett's to cancer. These patients need periodic endoscopic surveillance. If biopsies show no dysplasia, surveillance endoscopy can be performed less frequently. If dysplasia is present, an active, close watch and endoscopic or surgical strategies are applied before the condition evolves into a full blown carcinoma. There is an enormous effort among gastroenterologists and surgeons to find a tolerable way of resolving the Barrett's dilemma. Removing the affected mucosa by different endoscopic means is now available, as well as new surgical techniques that have improved the outcome of this pre-cancerous condition. Cancer of the esophagus has an increased incidence among Fosamax (a medication to treat osteoporosis) users. This highlights how cautious we need to be in taking any class of active medications because of their polarizing actions, helping on one hand and causing harm on the other, validating the concept that a life with little or no medications should be a universal aspiration.

Cancer of the Uterine Cervix: This was at one time the leading cause of death among women. The Papanicolau test dramatically changed its incidence. This test is usually performed in sexually active women or females that have reached 21 years of age, typically is carried annually for three consecutive tests and then after considering individual factors. The test is aimed to discover cell changes in the uterine cervix, which are usually caused by the human papillomaviruses (HPV) in sexually active woman. Early detection is usually life-saving. Immunization with two available HPV vaccines may confer partial protection against infection. Because the vaccines have been proven to be more effective in females before they have engaged in sexual activities, there is an ongoing controversy about vaccinating children at an early age, especially on religious and moral grounds. It is better for parents to discuss all concerns about HPV vaccine in children with a pediatrician.

Cancer of the Breast: There are 192,000 new cases diagnosed in the US every year and 40,000 will die from it. Males can be also affected but in very low proportion (1900 cases a year and 440 deaths). Mammogram is an imaging technique that has proved to be valuable in screening for cancer of the breast. The recommendation of the National Cancer Institute is for females over the age of forty to have a mammogram every one to two years. It should be emphasized that no test precludes a clinical examination of the breast by a competent physician. Recent studies by the US Prevention Services Task Force showed that patients between the ages of 40 and 50 develop breast cancer at a lower rate than those above 50. As a result they recommended for the younger females not to undergo routine mammograms. This produced a justifiable popular uproar. The commotion produced by their recommendations was such that the US government decided not to implement them. This decision was political and not based on science. Overscreening also carries some risks, like unnecessary surgery, increased exposure to radiation and the consequences of acting on a false positive or false negative result. Dr. Susan Love, the author of *Dr Susan Love's Breast Book* and a breast cancer surgeon at the UCLA's David Geffen School of Medicine, wrote about spacing mammograms in patients under 50, "They finally bring us into line with everyone else in the world. They are based on data, as opposed to wishful thinking." The recommendations did not apply to women at high risk (such as strong family history, those who started menstruating at an early age, late pregnancies, and previous suspicious biopsies). The actuarial data is clear: women under the age of 50 have a 1.4 percent chance of getting breast cancer, whereas those over 50 have a 2.4 percent chance and over 60, 3.4 percent. Mammograms have fewer false results in older women because of the texture of their breasts. Younger women have more aggressive cancers, which mean that early detection is desirable. On the other hand, we may be over-treating by removing a slow growing cancer, but this appears to be a non-argument since there is no way to know how cancers may behave. Some doctors and institutions are adamant interventionists, while others advocate caution before embarking on certain diagnostic or treatment modalities. The lack of consensus among physicians complicates the road to follow in breast cancer prevention. The value of mammograms in saving lives is incontrovertible. New techniques to improve the diagnostic yield of imaging studies are being developed. Digital mammography allows the storage of the image in the computer but is similar in results to conventional mammograms. MRIs (Magnetic Resonance Imaging) and PETs (Positron Emission Tomography) are currently being evaluated. Ultrasound of the breast is complementary and helps to decrease false positive results. The detection of some genetic alterations, like the BCR1 and BCR2 genes, that may be present in 10 percent of the people, has been a definitive preventative advance since they serve as markers for the possible development of a malignancy.

Women at high risk of developing cancer may benefit from the use of Raloxifen (a medication used for osteoporosis) and Tamoxifen (an antiestrogen medication). Certain breast cancer cells need estrogen to grow and Tamoxifen, an estrogen antagonist, has shown that it can prolong life in patients that had a cancer removed and are estrogen receptor positive and also prevent its appearance. If this were to be confirmed it would represent a very important therapeutic progress.

Exercise may preclude and obesity facilitates the appearance of breast cancer. These two areas deserve further scrutiny to make more definitive recommendations.

The use of estrogen replacement, which was so popular for many decades, was clearly a contributing factor in the development of breast cancer. The incidence of this condition decreased by 15 percent in post-menopausal women when the FDA sent an advisory notice to physicians and women stopped using it. And yet, recent reports showed that estrogen may prevent cancer of the breast in patients who had a hysterectomy. This subject was so confusing that Gail Collins, the editorialist of the *New York Times* asked doctors to "please make up your mind."

Melanoma and other skin cancers: Dermatological examination should be performed yearly either by a competent internist or a dermatologist. Visual examination can be helped by the use of a dermatoscope, a very simple instrument which magnifies a suspicious lesion, illuminating the area without reflecting light.

Decades ago it was fashionable to get a tan and it was a widespread practice to 'fry' under the sun without any protection. Cocoa butter and other oils were used to beautify the color of the skin, enhancing the aggression of the sun's rays; now we know better and yet there are millions chasing the sun to improve their looks. Sun exposure is also responsible for other types of skin cancer such as squamous and basal cell carcinoma. This year 60,000 new cases will be diagnosed with skin cancer and 48,000 will die from this condition. This is unacceptable because clothing protection, avoiding sun exposure and the use of lotions (which became popular after 1962) can halt the appearance of this dreadful condition. Tanning beds may also induce the appearance of melanoma and yet this tanning modality is more popular than ever.

Diabetes: Secondary prevention is achieved by diagnosing a pre-diabetic state. In the past diabetes (DM) was classified as insulin dependent and non-insulin dependent. Today DM is classified as type I, characterized by insulin deficiency and type II, where there is insulin resistance, impaired insulin secretion and excessive hepatic glucose production.

There are different means to diagnose a predisposition to DM, such as an abnormal fasting glucose or an impaired glucose tolerance test, of course before symptoms arise.

There are close to 10 million people affected with this condition in the US alone, requiring medical attention and using vast amounts of medical resources. Early diagnosis and lifestyle and eating pattern changes are part of the first line of prevention

Hypertension: Is categorized in two stages. The first is pre-hypertension, a stage that warns that the individual may be at risk to move to the more serious true hypertension. Readings between 120/80 to 139/89 describe the first category. Above 140/90 is considered established hypertension. The first number is called systolic blood pressure and measures the force of the blood after the heart contracts. The second number is called diastolic blood pressure and reflects the force after the heart relaxes. High blood pressure is called the silent killer because it may only manifest when it has produced end organ damage. Secondary prevention is simply achieved by measuring the blood pressure at different intervals. If it is consistently within normal limits, normal readings can be spaced. Hypertension requires early therapeutic intervention because sustained high blood pressure ends up injuring the heart, the kidneys, the brain and other organs.

Heart Disease: Determining risk assists in outlining a prevention strategy. Obesity, cocaine use, family history, diabetes, smoking, hypertension and sedentary life and weight are definitive threats to the heart. Basic prevention tests include measuring lipids and the High Sensitive C-Reactive Protein. Abnormal results call for aggressive diagnostic intervention. Heart disease has an ample range of manifestations from none until it hits, thus the striking manifestation of cardiac arrest in otherwise 'normal-appearing individuals' to total limitation of physical activity. Prevention is possible in the majority of cases, even for those who have a familial or genetic component.

Glaucoma: This is a condition that is produced by a rise in pressure of the eye fluid that can affect the optic nerve and result in significant loss of vision and blindness. To be sure, increased eye pressure is not glaucoma but increased pressure may damage the optic nerve. Once the damage is produced, the vision cannot be restored; that is why early measurement of eye pressure is so important.

Tooth disease: Tooth decay and periodontal disease produced by specific bacterial infections are prevented by sound oral hygiene and assistance by dental professionals. This is important because the mouth is the first part of the digestive system and as such, when impaired, may be the site of entrance of many disease conditions.

Oral cancer: Early detection and early treatment may dramatically reduce the mortality and morbidity associated with this condition. The survival rate on those diagnosed on the early stages is 82 percent and only 28 for late diagnosis. It takes only few minutes to make a thorough examination of the oral cavity, but you need to make sure that your doctor does not neglect this part of the body during a physical examination, something which they often do. Smoking, chewing tobacco and exposing your lips to the sun are definitive risk factors.

Infection Prevention: Infections can be prevented with simple measures, easy to postulate but difficult to adhere to. HIV is an example. Safe sex practices are difficult to enact because there are multiple factors such as socioeconomic status, availability of counselors, cultural and psychological dynamics and education. AIDS is a condition where opportunistic infections are common, as with any other immunodeficiency disorders. Other sexually transmitted conditions like gonorrhea, chlamydia, herpes genitalis, human papillomavirus, genital warts, pelvic inflammatory disease, thricomoniasis and vaginitis are preventable first by abstinence, second by safe sexual practices and third by early medical intervention. One example is the application of a vaccine against the papilloma virus, which is the precursor of cervical uterine cancer. Microbicides and female-barrier methods have been shown to be effective if properly applied. Flu, tuberculosis, nosocomial infections (which kill thousands in hospital settings), pneumococcal pneumonia, and all infections in general can be greatly reduced by limiting exposure, utilizing proper sanitary control, vaccines and enforcing safe hygienic measures.

Stroke Prevention: This condition is produced by the lack of blood to the brain, either by a blockage from a blood clot or by a hemorrhage, Strokes affect 600,000 persons a year, and there are 4 million stroke survivors with residual damage from cognitive to motor impairment of different degrees. The two main causes of a 'brain attack' are atrial fibrillation, an irregular rhythm of the heart that facilitates seeding of a clot, which may migrate to the brain and a blockage of the carotid artery, which is the main supplier of oxygen to the organ. Both atrial fibrillation and carotid artery blockage are easy to detect and their diagnoses are the mainstay for secondary prevention. Atrial fibrillation is first treated with medications and if uncontrolled, warfarin, an anticoagulant, is given to avoid clot formation. Carotid stenosis of a significant degree is treated by removal of a plaque or fatty deposit by endarterectomy, a surgical procedure that consists of removing the material that may be obstructing the flow in an artery.

4

In contrast to the above conditions, there are others that are not specifically preventable, such as:

Cancer of the Pancreas and other cancers
Alzheimer's
Blood Disorders
Endocrine Disorders
Rheumatoid Arthritis
Osteoporosis
Sexual Dysfunction
Tuberculosis of the Adrenal Gland

Cancer of the Pancreas and other cancers: Cancer of the pancreas is a dreadful condition that even when diagnosed already has a poor prognosis, in contrast with other cancers with a better outlook if diagnosed early.

There are no tumor markers that can alert us that a malignant pancreatic tumor is about to develop; rather, abnormal markers signal that a tumor is already present. Markers help to manage a condition, not to diagnose it. Risk markers are a different story. These are alterations or mutations in specific genes, that piece of DNA that is passed from parents to their offspring, and may alert that certain cancer is likely to occur. A typical example is the BRCA 1 and BRCA2 markers that indicate a predisposition to hereditary breast or ovarian cancer. These tests cost thousands of dollars and are not done as part of a routine checkup but rather reserved for females and males with a strong, unequivocal family history of breast and ovarian cancer. A negative result means that the person does not have familial susceptibility to acquire those conditions but not that they cannot develop them. There is an ongoing effort to identify risk indicators for carcinoma of the pancreas and others.

These conditions humble us and show that in spite of all we know about the human body, we still know very little. Cancer of the pancreas is as elusive as a bird. I remember so many of these patients, their despair, the angst of family and friends and the efforts to stay alive. Amanda R. a long-time, dear patient of mine realized how hopeless I felt for not being able to help and gave me comfort. "That's OK doc," she told me. "I am at peace with myself and accept that it is time to go, I have my faith and my faith is my strength, I have lived a full life; thanks for all you have done for me."

Alzheimer's: This condition appears mainly in people over the age of 60 and is a dreaded disease that relentlessly attacks the memory and thought process, impairing the ability to carry out simple, daily, routine activities. About 4 million people have Alzheimer's disease in the US. Survival average is three to four years in individuals over the age of 80 and longer if younger. There is no sound preventive advice, although anecdotes are abundant. Some claim that polyglots or those engaged in mentally stimulating activities or who are socially active may have a decreased incidence of the disease, all unproven assertions. Once Alzheimer's takes full possession of the individual, their fate is in the hands of their loved ones. There is a colossal effort by medical institutions and by other organizations to conquer the disease. There has been some progress in understanding how the loss of neurons, amyloid deposits and plaque formation produce degenerative changes but none have translated in a meaningful way to manage the disease. Cognitive stimulation, mental exercises, music, pet therapy, social interaction, learning another language, and keeping active till the end of life are measures that have been advocated with no complete efficacy but since they are innocuous they can be instituted without harm.

Blood Disorders: During routine blood examinations it is not unusual to detect certain blood disorders. These are diagnostic and not preventive tests. For example, if laboratory results suggest chronic myelocitic leukemia there is no way of knowing how long the condition has been present. The bone marrow is the factory and distribution center of blood elements and it may be affected in its function by radiation, drugs, toxins and other environmental factors to prevent the onset of leukemia, lymphoma, and other blood disorders. Lead, mercury, vitamins, minerals and radiation are toxic once they pass certain thresholds.

Endocrine Disorders: Adrenal, thyroid, pituitary, bone parathyroid, and gonads are affected with degenerative, infectious, malignant or inflammatory changes. Many of the causes are unknown, while others have been identified.

Osteoporosis :May be prevented or slowed but not avoided by staying slim and fit, being exposed to sunlight to enhance absorption of vitamin D, getting enough calcium in the diet, and exercising.

Sexual dysfunction: Is ameliorated by avoiding drugs or prescription medication known to alter potency and libido but there is subset where the cause is unknown and we cannot do too much to help.

Tuberculosis of the adrenal gland: Is avoided by sanitary control, similar to all types of infections, and yet they may appear in spite of those efforts.

Rheumatoid arthritis: This condition affects about 1.3 million people in the US. It can be a devastating disease with significant health and social implications. There are no primary or secondary preventive measures and yet as with this and as many others diseases even if not scientifically proven a healthy lifestyle may be a disincentive for it appearance.

Nature is our friend; it provides for all our needs. It is only when we tamper with or abuse it that it becomes the enemy.

5

Tertiary prevention refers to all the things patients and health professionals can do once a **condition is established**. The following is a list of the most common conditions that can be positively affected by tertiary prevention:

Diabetes
Hypertension
Cardiovascular Disease
Stroke
Cancer

Diabetes: Metabolic Syndrome (MS) refers to a component of diabetes where the patient develops insulin resistance. Reversal of MS is not easy but possible. Unfortunately modifying triglycerides or High Density Lipoprotein does not improve insulin action. But it appears that interventions to target abdominal obesity and/or impaired fasting glucose may be of benefit. Weight reduction and exercise are the two most important factors in this equation. Although appetite suppressants may temporarily help to achieve these goals, the most desirable measure is lifestyle modification. Waist circumference reduction is the most favorable indicator to predict clinical improvement. Abdominal girth is attributable to inactivity, independent of Body Mass Index. There are specific pharmacological interventions to reduce insulin sensitization, which are outside the scope of this book.

Hypertension: As a response to prolonged hypertension, the heart needs to pump blood more vigorously and the left ventricle becomes enlarged, like when the arm muscles increase their mass and strength after prolonged periods of exercise. In the case of the heart, as desirable as it may appear to be at first glance, it is not so, because when the resistance is permanent, as it is in the case of hypertension, the heart is not able to handle the load and cardiac insufficiency ensues. It follows that hypertension control is mandatory. The pharmacological interventions are usually successful, although none of the medications are exempt from side effects. Managing the blood pressure without medications is, again, like climbing the Everest. In my case, I was taking two antihypertensive medications with good results. My weight was 180 pounds, mildly elevated. I decided to eat judiciously, reduce fat intake and salt and increase vegetable and fruit consumption. At the same time I changed my exercise routine and started swimming one hour a day four to five times a week and aerobic and resistance training two to three days a week, in addition started on 3000 mg of fish oil daily. My weight went down to 167 and my blood pressure without medications today is as on average around 115/72.

Cardiovascular Disease: Once atherosclerosis is established, which is the main pathological process leading to coronary artery disease, stroke and peripheral vascular disease, it is time to take action to reduce the unrewarding consequences that it brings. Atherosclerosis is usually asymptomatic for a long period. Tobacco use, obesity, abnormal blood lipids, excessive alcohol, too much salt, hypertension and a sedentary life are the wrongdoers, the villains of this story.

Risk prediction in cardiovascular disease is dependent on race, gender, socioeconomic status, family history, associated medical conditions, lifestyle and ethnicity. Some of these factors we cannot modify, but correct identification allows vigorous early preventive intervention. Certain medications like oral contraceptives, licorice, nonsteroidal anti-inflammatory drugs, amphetamines, cocaine, erythropoietin, cyclosporins and steroid are known to raise the blood pressure, therefore some of them need to be eliminated altogether and others adjusted to the right amount. Other aspects, seldom discussed and many times ignored, are the personal, psychosocial, occupational and environmental factors that can influence the heart, the blood pressure and all other diseases.

Stroke: Once the pharmacological treatment and the rehabilitation strategy have been clearly formulated by the professionals in charge of the care of a patient who has suffered a cerebrovascular accident, it is important to apply simultaneous tertiary measures to reduce recurrence and to improve the quality of life. At the risk of being excessively repetitive, I will once more list the elements consistent with a positive lifestyle modification: weight control, no tobacco or excessive alcohol, enhanced physical activity, stress reduction, strict overview of current medications since many may inadvertently cause symptoms that wrongly are attributable to stroke, such as antidepressive, tranquilizers, antihypertensives and other drugs, a situation that we have seen again and again.

Cancer: As dreaded as the word sounds not all cancers are necessarily fatal. Furthermore, some that were lethal not too long ago may be cured by early intervention. An example is chronic myeloid leukemia (CML), once a death sentence and now a manageable condition with the use of Gleevek, a medication developed by Drs. Brian J. Druker, Charles L. Swayers and Nicholas B. Lydon. This disease killed all patients about one year after onset, even when alfa Interferon, the only available medication at that time was instituted. If an author of a novel wanted to create a life situation where a physician tells a patient, "You have one year to live," this was it. Gleevek specifically targets cancer cells, leaving healthy ones alone by blocking an enzyme responsible for the uncontrolled growth of cancer cells. I applied this medication in a patient of mine who had a gastric stromal tumor detected by upper endoscopy in 1991, when this medication was in its early infancy. Up to that moment we gastroenterologists, had seen tumors disappear after surgical, radiation or strong chemo treatments but we had never seen a tumor vanish by just taking a medication. Gleevek has some occasional serious secondary effects, but the potential for cure outweighs the undesirable effects. The main side effect is the cost: 32,000 dollars a year.

6

Is there an Ideal Daily Medication Routine?

The pharmaceutical companies want all of us to take daily medications in order to prevent the onset of different calamities. At the same time if they succeed their coffers would increase by geometric proportions. Some of their advice is sound while other is unfortunate.

Aspirin: The old adage that an apple a day keeps the doctor away was simple and a sensible one. After all, an apple contains vitamins, antioxidants and good nutritional value. As things go, this allegory may soon be replaced by an aspirin a day keeps the doctor away, because aspirin certainly has definite health benefits.

The question once posed by the World Health Organization was: Does long term treatment with aspirin reduce cardiovascular risk?

The answer is a qualified yes. Multiple research papers and epidemiological studies show that compared to placebo, aspirin was associated with a 32 percent reduction in myocardial infarction (MI) and a non-significant increase in the risk of stroke in men. Paradoxically, in a 10 year study females were not benefited for prevention of MI but it lower the risk of stroke. Other data published in the journal *Circulation* showed the benefits of baby aspirin in a cohort of female patients over the age of 65. Because females have different presentation, diagnoses and treatments when it comes to cardiovascular disease, new evidence–based guidelines are needed for the prevention of Coronary Heart Disease (CHD). Post-menopausal females should avoid hormonal replacement and Vitamin E, whose beneficial effects are questionable.

The shortcoming of this recommendation is that aspirin doubles the risk of gastrointestinal bleeding. Of 1000 patients, one to two may bleed from the gastrointestinal tract, which means that on a few occasions the benefits may be outweighed by this undesirable side effect. Yet identifying those who are at risk of MI and recommending aspirin, taking into consideration age, sex and associated conditions may minimize the absolute excess risk.

In general a low dose aspirin (75 mg/day), which represents ¼ of regular aspirin, is recommended for all patients at high risk of developing CHD, providing that their blood pressure is under control, they are not allergic to the compound and they have no history of gastrointestinal hemorrhage.

Finasteride: Finasteride and duasteride, two medications that minimize the testosterone effect on the prostate, are known to cut the risk of prostate cancer by 25 percent. Present conventional wisdom is that they should be prescribed by a urologist after meticulous discussion about their pros and cons.

Statins: It is now being recommended to take statins to prevent plaque formation, even in those who have a normal cholesterol level and normal ratio between the good and bad cholesterol. Yet undesirable side effects may prevent many from taking them and **in all cases lifestyle changes may be a better approach**. Those who have had a CAD incident and those with abnormal cholesterol values may need to take them to prevent another attack.

Tamoxifen and Raloxifene: The first one is an antagonist of the estrogen receptor in the breast and the second is a selective estrogen modulator. Both have been shown to decrease the incidence of breast cancer by 50 percent. Tamoxifen is currently used to prevent a recurrence of this malignancy and not as a preventative. Raloxifene is used to treat osteoporosis. As with almost all active medications, they are not free of undesirable side effects. Raloxifene produces clots and strokes in a few cases, and tamoxifen has been linked to cancer of the uterine endometrium. Therefore it should be used in selective cases only.

Fish oil: Contains Omega-3 fatty acids and other substances with strong anti-inflammatory effects. Multiple studies have shown that at a dose of 1 to 3 grams a day it lowers cholesterol, decreases hypertension, decreases depression and suicidal ideation, prevents the progression of CAD, and it may decrease the incidence of breast, colon and prostate cancer. Ideally, fish oil should be obtained by eating fish, but since they may contain pollutants such as mercury, dioxin, chlordane and PCBs fish oil tablets may substitute fish providing that the purification and manufacturing of the tablets is performed under rigorous conditions. Fish oil at high doses may increase the risk of bleeding, stroke and glycemic control, but not at the recommended dose.

Vitamins: The regular American diet contains more than enough vitamins to satisfy the nutritional requirements of the human body. Vitamins C, A, E and folic acid in **large doses may end up being more harmful than beneficial.** Scientifically speaking, there is no reason for those eating a balanced diet to take them, although millions of us are taking multivitamins at an adjusted dose, not exceeding daily requirements.

Nutritional Supplements: They are by far bogus in their claims. None of them have proven to boost brain function, enhance libido, heighten stamina, improve flexibility, regulate bowel function, prevent cancer, improve sleep and in general advance our bodily functions. What they do, besides the expense, is to give the illusion of achieving wellbeing by their strong placebo effect but as with other illusions, the effects are ephemeral. As with vitamins, they should not replace other sound measures to be and stay well. The confusion arises by equating deficiencies when none exist with beneficial effects. B vitamins deficiency is associated with age-related neurocognitive disorders and only those who are deficient benefit from their intake. Calcium may be taken as a supplement as an extra effort to maintain normal levels in certain cases, for example when the person has little exposure to sunlight, a necessary prerequisite for vitamin D synthesis that enhances calcium absorption. Vitamins and nutritional supplements are indicated in specific cases like pregnancy (where folic acid is needed) or certain anemias (where iron is a must) or alcoholics (who are folate deficient by the nature of the disease).

Extrapolating experimental results in animals to humans is not prudent; they should rather be the foundation to conduct clinical trials. Folic acid (the synthetic form of folates) is known to decrease homocysteine levels, which are associated with cardiovascular disease, and yet there are no clinical studies that show a decrease in CAD.

Green tea supporters claim that it can prevent cancer from their antioxidant properties. As hopeful as these assertions are, clinical studies have shown mixed results. Green tea contains caffeine and may produce insomnia and vitamin K may counteract with warfarin in those who need optimal anticoagulation effect. The list of unproven benefits of nutritional supplements in humans is extensive and caution is always required.

Taking herbs should be based on science. To pop several tablets a day is easier than to exercise or to eat judiciously. Critical thinking is essential; decisions should be based on objective data, validated experimentation and proven facts. We need to dispose of fantasies, illusions and myths and replace them with positive actions. Becoming an active participant, based on knowledge and not fantasies, in your decisions and actions will be empowering.

7

In essence:

A "polypill" consisting of a statin, three antihypertensive agents at half doses, baby aspirin and folic acid has been proposed as a way of avoiding heart problems and stroke. The risk reduction was estimated to be 88 percent for CAD and 80 percent for stroke. **This is a work in progress because further evidence supporting the use of combination therapy is needed.** The idea of providing people a "polypill" to enhance adherence to treatment and avoid inadequate dosages was developed as a means of mass treatment. This is an interesting concept, **still in its early infancy.**

For the moment the sensible thing to do, for **certain age groups and specific conditions,** is to take a baby aspirin daily, 1 to 3 grams of fish oil and one multivitamin a day. Other supplementation needs to be tailored to specific cases, but in all cases everybody should get advice from a physician before taking any type of drugs.

Chapter 9:

Whatever it takes:

The Role of Conventional and Alternative Medicine in Preserving Health.

The market for Alternative Medicine is vast and growing... This trend must be guided by scientific inquiry, clinical judgment, regulatory authority and shared decision-making.   David Eisenberg

1

About ten years ago I saw a 62 year old patient in my office who had problems swallowing first liquids and then solids. He had those complaints for more than one year. He saw a physician who adhered to Linus Pauling's precepts, who prescribed him with large doses of oral Vitamin C. Since he was getting progressively worse, he sought a second opinion. I performed an upper endoscopy which showed a fungated mass in the distal esophagus consistent with an adenocarcinoma, confirmed by multiple biopsies. He underwent a surgical resection of the tumor but died one year later from metastatic disease. I was appalled that his symptoms were ignored by his doctor and surprised that he had received Vitamin C as the sole form of treatment. Dr. Pauling was a brilliant scientist, a political activist and a remarkable human being. He received two Nobel Prizes, one for chemistry and one for his peace efforts. His works on quantum mechanics were impressive. Late in his career he started advocating the use of large amounts of Vitamin C for all kinds of illnesses. All of his assertions about the use of vitamin C were proven to be wrong. He had his allies and his enemies. In 1985 Dr. Moertel, a respected gastroenterologist from the Mayo Clinic, had an open confrontation with Dr. Pauling, accusing him of scientific incompetence and equating his postulates regarding the use of certain diets and vitamins with quackery.

Dr. Pauling went so far as advocating vitamin C be taken either orally or intravenously to prevent atherosclerosis and relieve angina pectoris. His legacy became tainted by his insistence on the therapeutic value of vitamin C, claims that had been counterintuitive to what we know about cancer. As a consequence my patient, and probably many others, by adhering to Pauling's predicaments, were hurt by delaying or ignoring valid treatments.

About the same time I saw a 50 year old patient who had multiple large abdominal masses. His more prominent symptoms were abdominal pain, ascites and weight loss. A work-up revealed primary malignant mesothelioma, a very aggressive cancer with a very poor prognosis. Several experimental treatments were attempted by the oncologist but with no response. In spite of his dismal outlook he had a positive attitude and told us that he was determined to do his utmost to fight the disease. He sought help from cancer support groups, family and friends, enrolled in yoga classes and much to our surprise, he got better. He lived three more years, surpassing the life expectancy for this kind of patient.

In the first case ignoring what conventional medicine had to offer precipitated a fatal outcome and in the other a strong will, determination and emotional fortitude helped in extending life.

Many patients choose to seek help outside the current medical system and resort to unconventional means of health maintenance. This approach is known as alternative or complementary medicine, and it is viewed by many physicians as dangerous because some patients postpone visits to the doctor's office, delaying timely diagnosis, aggravating an existing illness or making it irreversible.

Medicine is an organized system of information based on the scientific method; something becomes certain when it is reproducible and verifiable, which is conducive to rational impartiality. Medicine, as it is known today, evolved as a departure from traditional approaches that counted intuition, good judgment and experience as the basis of its practice. The contribution of the scientific method to the knowledge of body structure, function and disease has been phenomenal.

Medicine is also an art that entails the use of creative imagination, experience and common sense.

Being a combination of science and art, medicine practiced in Western civilization is a solid discipline with a fundamental role of the preservation and restoration of health. Its goal is to prevent and conquer disease. The enthusiasm generated after the sixteenth century by the advent of science led us to believe that knowing the descriptive and topographic aspects of anatomy and the physiological and pathophysiological aspects of our body would suffice to control disease. If factor A produced disease B, controlling or eliminating factor A would eliminate disease B. This concept became entrenched in the practice of medicine. It took centuries to realize that the restoration of health was not simply achieved by removing external agents, and this brought back the concept that mind and spirit influence disease and recovery. Since mind and spirit are connected to the mystery of life, they were out of reach to the scientist, and this created a vacuum in the understanding of wellbeing and sickness. The frustration that this produced made some redefine the concept of health. Health was no longer the lack of physical symptoms or abnormal findings but rather a state of physical and emotional wellbeing.

The realization that in spite of new techniques and advanced treatment modalities, millions of Americans had unresolved health problems puzzled epidemiologists and health professionals. More than half of the population in the United States is using prescribed medications, in addition to the millions using non-prescription drugs and yet the incidence of chronic conditions such as arthritis, respiratory ailments, cardiovascular disease, lower back pain and headaches is similar today to what it was several decades ago. A survey from 1972 showed that only 6% of the population reported high energy and had no emotional or physical complaints. Robust health appeared to be the domain of the very few.

It is not surprising, then, that this created dissatisfaction with the medical system and the need to look for alternative ways for health preservation and restoration.

2

Holistic Medicine is an unorganized medical system opposed to structured medicine, developed as a way to treat the patient as a whole, taking into consideration physical, emotional, psychological and social components.

The basis of the holistic practice is the integration of body, mind and environment to treat and prevent disease. Holistic practitioners put emphasis on treating conditions in which present medical technology is of limited efficacy, such as degenerative diseases like arthritis or other common ailments like hypertension, cardiovascular diseases, diabetes and sexual impotence. They integrate orthodox and non-orthodox approaches and put emphasis on education and self-responsibility.

The non-conventional 'curative' techniques include mental imagery, which was one of the first systematic emotional interventions for the treatment of cancer patients, healing through music, lifestyle modification, relaxation and stress management, yoga, self-hypnosis and mental induction. Transcendental meditation, introduced by the Yogi Maharishi Mahesh, encompasses multiple techniques to gain emotional stability, energy, happiness, self control, self enlightening and inner peace. Studies have claimed reduction blood pressure, helping insomniacs and asthma sufferers, controlling anxiety and decreasing smoking and excessive alcohol intake. Some of these claims have been validated in reputable scientific institutions, while others are tantamount to quackery. The pharmacopeia of holistic medicine is extensive and is based on the use of natural substances, some proved to be effective and others completely useless.

It is difficult to make a general assertion about the value of Holistic Medicine because it means different things to different people and being a dislocated structure makes it difficult to evaluate.

3

According to Chinese medicine, the Chi or life energy is the essence of a healthy body. Disruption of the Chi leads to illness. The application of **Tai Chi**, which is a combination of martial arts techniques, restores the chi and consequently assures good health and longevity. It is a respected method of health restoration and prevention practiced by millions all over the world. It is embedded in principles of Chinese philosophy of the fusion of the Ying and Yang. It offers a state of calmness and relaxation that relieves physical stress. The Mayo Clinic endorses with certain qualifications the use of this technique as a non-expensive way of helping or eliminating anxiety and depression; improving flexibility, balance and muscle strength; reducing falls; lowering blood pressure; relieving cardiovascular fitness in older adults; increasing endurance, agility and energy; relieving chronic pain and improving overall feelings of wellbeing. Tai-Chi classes may be found in the YWCA, senior centers, health clubs and community centers, among others. Once or twice a week sessions of Tai Chi may be enough to provide long-lasting comfort. **None other than the prestigious *New England Journal of Medicine* has published a paper in August 2010 stating that this method may effectively help relieve fibromyalgia, a condition difficult to treat by conventional methods.**

Acupuncture is based on traditional Chinese medicine and has been practiced for thousands of years. It consists in the insertion of fine needles into the skin at specially designated points with the concept that certain points of the body can be stimulated to restore and maintain health. It is used for the treatment of ulcers, back pain, headaches, arthritis, and hypertension and as an anesthetic during childbirth and different types of surgery. It application evokes a stimulation or inhibition of the autonomic nervous system, thus its therapeutic effect. The list of conditions helped by acupuncture is extensive and includes practically all common diseases known to man. Performed by qualified persons, it is practically free of side effects, providing that the needles are disposable, sterile and non-toxic. It appeal is undeniable since it is based on maintaining the balance between the yin and the yang, the passive and the active principles of the mind and body, which is seen as an interconnected web. By stimulating certain points, acupuncture may relieve pain and various other conditions. It is practiced by doctors, dentists and other practitioners and is widely popular in the United States, attested by the thousands of dedicated places. More than one million people are said to have acupuncture every year.

The NCCAM has funded many studies to learn whether acupuncture works for specific health conditions such as chronic low-back pain, headaches and osteoarthritis of the knee. These studies are still in progress. The expectation goes from optimism from the believers such as the National Institute of Health who claimed that there is enough evidence that acupuncture is what it claims to be to the American Medical Association, which advises prudence and caution when using acupuncture.

Rolfing, named after its developer Ida Rolf, consists of deep, often painful massage to reestablish the natural state of the body and provide balance. There is no scientific data to validate its usefulness. As with other procedures like acupressure and massage, it is being tested to assess its validity as a therapeutic technique.

Psychic healing refers to the power of the mind to restore health and prevent illness by the use of the mind-body connection to enhance optimal body function. It includes the use of music, art and dance to manage disease and others like prayer and meditation to resolve stress and conflicts that may be interfering with healing.

Homeopathy consists of miniscule administration of substances that mimic the disease. Hahnemann, the father of homeopathy, claimed that cure proceeds to similarity ("like cures like principle"). Most analyses have concluded that there is little evidence to support homeopathy as an effective treatment for any specific condition, although there have been isolated randomized placebo-controlled trials and laboratory research that report positive effects of homeopathic remedies. During my practice I have seen some patients reporting beneficial results from their interaction with the homeopathic practitioner, but I have never seen any alleviation or cure in patients affected with organic conditions such as Inflammatory Bowel Disease, cancer or others.

Iridology is a diagnostic tool that looks at the color, shape and texture of the eye to formulate a diagnosis. It has no validity. **It is quackery or pseudo-science,** at best, and part of the techniques that naturopathic practitioners utilize.

4

Most of the alternative medicine techniques are unsupported by modern science. They are usually safe, but they carry the peril of halting the diagnosis and treatment of diseases that could be otherwise managed by conventional medicine.

Doctors need to understand that a large group of patients are favorably predisposed to alternative because of unhappiness or frustration with conservative medicine, while others feel an intellectual attraction for what alternative medicine offers or seek help out of desperation and as a last resort. Jorge, a 45 year old patient of mine with terminal pancreatic carcinoma in Los Angeles, visited a 'doctor' in San Diego who 'removed the cancer' from his abdomen. He gave the cancer to him, which looked like a piece of flesh. He had no visible scar; the 'doctor' healed the skin immediately. He felt great for few days. Jorge was mentally competent and coherent in every other aspect, demonstrating once more that the power of suggestion is strong and serves our defense mechanisms well. He died days later.

The part of alternative medicine that suggests lifestyle modification, positive thinking, minimizing environmental hazards and giving emotional and psychological support is welcome. But caution is needed; guidelines for alternative medicine are fussy and supervision by professional organizations non-existent. Fads are always a step away.

Primal Therapy, est, Transcendental Meditation and Lucid Dreaming are psychological techniques with different aims but with a common purpose: to achieve inner peace and empower a person to become a master of his emotions and by doing so become able to control angst, depression, and negative feelings and achieve a spiritual state conducive to physical and emotional wellbeing.

5

In summary: Although there is a place for Alternative Medicine, caution is required. Don't fall for narratives that create the illusion of achieving wellness through unorthodox methods. Don't postpone visiting a conventional doctor when your problems don't go away within a short period of time. Easy rhetoric and sophisms are appealing but misleading and flawed and may lead to fatal consequences. Deceiving practices are extremely common. The perpetrators are disguised as reputable physicians, medical institutions, pharmaceutical corporations, preachers, celebrities, and the media, among others. Avoid falling for misleading practices that will betray, maim or kill you.

Chapter 10

Clear Skies

The Environment Chapter

We cannot command Nature except by obeying her.   Francis Bacon

1

There is no discussion: the air we breathe and the water we drink are contaminated with undesirable pollutants. Plastic bottles, household cleaners, containers, detergents, preservatives, fertilizers, to name just a few, contain toxins that find the way to our body, producing serious health effects.

So let's turn an inconvenient truth in a convenient one. The more we know about environmental hazards, the more we can do to fight them.

The Environmental Protection Agency (EPA) has identified 187 pollutants, most of which cause cancer and reproductive and birth defects. Examples of toxic air pollutants include benzene, which is found in gasoline; perchlorethylene, which is emitted from some dry cleaning facilities and methylene chloride, a solvent and paint stripper used by a number of industries. Examples of other listed air toxins include dioxin, asbestos, toluene and metals such as cadmium, mercury, chromium and lead compounds.

Prolonged exposure to any of these may cause respiratory problems, neurological ailments, birth defects and other health problems. In addition, some toxic water or air pollutants such as mercury can deposit into soils or surface waters where they are taken up by plants and ingested by animals, eventually reaching us through the food chain.

We are exposed to toxic water or air pollutants by eating contaminated foods, breathing contaminated air, drinking water with toxins, ingesting edibles grown from contaminated soil, touching all types of infected surfaces, occupational exposure and by the use of cigarettes and recreational drugs.

I enjoy reading the newspaper in the morning while having breakfast. This ritual more than once becomes unpleasant when reading about all kinds of calamities. On the subject of pollution, in its December 8, 2009 edition the *New York Times* published an article about drinking water. Forty-nine million people have been drinking water that contained illegal concentrations of chemicals like arsenic, uranium (radioactive substance) and bacteria, causing millions of illnesses. In Ramsey, New Jersey, drinking water tests detected illegal concentrations of arsenic and a dry cleaning solvent, tetrachloroethylene, which has been linked to cancer. The problem is widespread, affecting almost every state in the Union. It is estimated that about 19 million people become ill each year from bacteria, viruses or parasites. The increasing incidence of prostate and breast cancer may be tied to water pollutants. In some areas the amount of radium detected in drinking water was 2,000 percent higher than the legal limit. In addition, a mother exposed to those hazards may transmit them to the baby to come, with nefarious consequences in the short and long run, like heart problems that may appear 50 years later. Annie Murphy Paul in her book *Origins: How The Nine Months Before Birth Shape the Rest of Our Lives* states that pregnant women who live in poverty with their dose of depression, anxiety, exposure to toxins, unhealthy eating and other bad habits, may bear children who may end up having severe health and social problems. Prenatal development affects individuals for the rest of their lives and may be passed from generation to generation in the form of diabetes, heart disease and/or mental illness.

In spite of the efforts of the EPA in decreasing and controlling the amount of pollutants released into the air, it remains a colossal problem with no solution in sight.

Santiago, Chile, is one of the worst affected cities in the world in terms of polluted air. It is built against the backdrop of the Andes and the smog most of the time has nowhere to go. When air quality is at its worst, admissions to hospitals for migraines and headaches increase significantly. *The Journal of Epidemiology and Community Health* reported a study showing that obese people react to air pollution with an increase in blood pressure, which compounds their other health problems.

Fighting air pollution is a collective responsibility, and we all need to be accountable for the present environmental disaster as much as industries, the government, institutions and the corporate world.

These are EPA recommendations when ozone is expected to be unhealthy:

Conserve electricity and set your air conditioner at higher temperature.
Choose a cleaner commute.
Bicycle to work or to errands when possible.
Defer use of gasoline-powered lawn and garden equipment for later in the day, or for days when the air quality is better.
Refuel cars and trucks after dusk.
Limit engine idling.
Get regular engine tune-ups and car maintenance checks (especially spark plugs).
Avoid spilling gas and don't "top off" the tank. Replace gas tank cap tightly.
Properly dispose of household paints, solvents and pesticides. Store these items in airtight containers.
Paint with a brush, not a sprayer.

In addition, to reduce or prevent unhealthy levels of particle pollution, the EPA recommends the following actions:

> Reduce or eliminate fireplace and wood stove use.
> Avoid using gas-powered lawn and garden equipment.
> Avoid burning leaves, trash and other materials.
> Use household, workshop, and garden chemicals in a
> way that keeps evaporation to a minimum, or try to
> delay using them when poor quality air is forecast.
> Replace your car's air filter and oil regularly.

The water pollutants may appear at the source--rivers, streams, lakes and ocean--or may be contaminated by industries and agricultural practices. Runoff from major urban areas and agricultural fields produces potential harmful chemical pollution. Nutrient pollution is the largest problem facing US coastal waters, as it alters the balance of nature by poisoning shellfish, harming algal blooms, destroying coral reef and killing mammals and seabirds.

Add to this the presence of sex hormones, painkillers and/or anticholesterol drugs and other pharmaceuticals, as was shown in treated drinking waters, and the problem becomes overbearing. The waste we produce is coming back to us and we have to upgrade treatment plans to prevent further damage to our health. The time is now.

An article published in *Consumer Reports* (December 2009) tested 19 different types of canned foods and found that almost all of them contain measurable amounts of Bisphenol A (BPA), which contaminates food from metal and, to a lesser degree, plastic containers.

2

I became a physician long before the era when the environment surrounding all of us was a real concern. Only some occupational hazards were recognized as a problem: coal miners got coal worker's pneumoconiosis; silicon workers, silicosis; moldy hay produced farmer's lung and so forth. Since these conditions were confined to a small group of workers, the preoccupation with them was also confined to only a few.

We don't have a good explanation for why some people in a determined area get sick with cancer while others are able to escape this fatality. Chile and Japan have a significant incidence of cancer of the stomach compared, for example, to the United States. Liver cancer is common in the Philippines; lung and breast cancer are more common in developed countries; risk for esophageal cancer has been noted to be higher in a brewery in Denmark, reaching tragic proportions without a good explanation. Sometimes we can explain why there are clusters of cancer in certain populations, while in other cases our best explanation is that its randomness is due to 'bad luck.'

At the beginning of the century cancers of unknown origin were attributed to viruses. Present concerns like pollutants, chemicals and other toxins did not enter our minds until decades later. We knew that certain cancers were familial or had a genetic component but we could not specifically identify them until later. The reason that some people were not resistant to certain diseases was explained in a vague way by saying that they probably had an immune disorder which now we can define better by the discovery of the role of T & B lymphocytes and their subpopulations. These are cells that originate in the bone marrow and are distributed to different parts of the body, where they exert a protection against viruses, infections, tumor cells and allergens by either evoking an immune response or the formation of antibodies, helped at times by other cells in the body like macrophages and NK, or natural killer, cells.

Although today we know so much more than we knew then, for instance, that our internal composition is shaped by what we ingest, by bodily motion or by our emotional life, we still don't have an explanation for the frequent question of cancer patients of "why me?". Most likely there is a combination of all the factors mentioned above that may produce a mutation in the DNA sequence, increasing the expression of oncogenes (which facilitates cancer) or deletion of tumor suppressor genes (which stops cancer) or a combination of both. These two elements are largely influenced by what we ingest, in the form of food or chemicals, or to what we are exposed. It follows then that the polluted environment is a problem that needs to be addressed. In part it is being tackled by governmental agencies that oversee the safety and health of individuals; unfortunately, many industries oppose legislation to safeguard our wellbeing when it runs contrary to their financial interests. The problem is compounded by the disregard of some who look at environmental protection like a political problem, by those who use the earth as a source for an endless appetite for material things, irrespective of the damage to our natural reserves.

3

How can we help in keeping the skies blue and the waters clear? This is a question with a very simple answer. Be responsible and do your part: avoid wasteful consumption, don't patronize industries or corporations that disregard the beauty and the wellness of our natural world, do your part in maintaining the ecosystem intact, don't drive if you can walk, set the thermostat of your house at a reasonable temperature, use your own bag for groceries, consume to satisfy your needs and not lavishness, drive fuel efficient cars, practice opulence of the spirit and not the opulence of material things, avoid plastic containers, read the labels of what you eat and avoid those products that contain chemicals, invent a world of inner comfort and less external indulgence.

4

There is an ongoing debate between small groups of people who claim that environmental hazards are greatly exaggerated, not proven and a figment of the imagination from some who want to advance a political agenda. This is in opposition to science, which conclusively and unequivocally has shown that the contamination of the atmosphere is pervasive and its consequences nefarious. The effects of a polluted environment are here for everybody to see, and yet it is being ignored by those who are responsible for being the polluters. Just looking at who they are would suffice to make it clear where the truth lies. Let's take, for example, bisphenol A, or BPA, as it is commonly known. This substance was declared by the government of Canada to be toxic to human health and to the environment. As such it was banned from use in baby bottles and considered to be prohibited in other containers like cans. The Canadian chemical industry mounted a strong opposition to these regulations, happily without success, since it clearly affects a vital source of income for them and their stockholders. Who is also in favor of this ban? Medical societies see these pollutants as an endocrine disruptor that produces a large series of illnesses like infertility, malformations and cancers. Who is opposed? Industries with a material interest in the product. These conflicting interests plus the enormous amount of data about environmental toxins and other hazards indicates that we all need to become involved in this discussion and demand to live in a world where the present risks and dangers can be minimized.

Chapter 11

The Pastoral Life

The Transformational Chapter

To be the masters of our destiny, our heath and our spirit, we need a profound cultural, social and personal renovation.

We are coming to the end of the book. Before we depart, we need to discuss the steps that you need to take to change what appears to be an ominous fate. Trust me, you can do it. I understand that it won't be easy, if this were the case, we would not be in the position we are today. Just look around. How many people do you see who have lost their body flexibility? Their knees have given up. They cannot go up a flight of stairs. Some use a cane, others are in a wheelchair. Some are obese, others morbidly obese. They look tired. Come with me to a convalescent home. This is Susie; she is 72 years old, has diabetes and had a stroke two years ago that left her with a right side paralysis and slurred speech. Mary is also 72 she had severe osteoporosis and broke her hip twice. George is 78; his hands are so deformed from arthritis that he needs help to eat. The three of them have a long history of neglect, never attending to their health issues and little by little they became sick, dysfunctional and a burden to themselves and society.

Aging is part of our evolution, manifested by physical, mental and emotional changes. The skin loses elasticity, aging spots appear, the matrix of the skin becomes thin and the skin becomes dry. Modern life, with its high level of noise in the city, accelerates hearing loss, which usually starts in the seventies. Muscles, which reach full maturity in the second decade of life, without exercise lose mass and power before their time.

The quality of bone is established in younger years and its condition in later times reflects how one has used them. Use it or lose it. Osteoporosis appears early. Rigidity of the thoracic cage, which causes less efficient breathing is accelerated in sedentary people. The curvature of the spine gives a bowed appearance to some elderly people but those who remain physically active throughout their lives will not display this posture, even in their late 80s. The basal metabolism rate slowly reduces over the years, and the quantity of oxygen used by tissues varies from organ to organ. Changes at a cellular level ultimately reduce production of energy and working capacity.

Old people are more sensitive to the lack of oxygen, yet those who have been engaged in a regular exercise program throughout life will be less restricted than one who is sedentary. Sustained high blood pressure adds a load to the heart, adding to the slower contraction of the heart and the rigidity of the walls of the arteries. Repeated mini-strokes produce slow mental deterioration.

In this book we said over and over again that staying healthy is easy; all it takes is good nutrition, enhanced physical activity and stress reduction. But there are external forces hindering our desires to stay healthy. These forces are powerful and influence our behavior relentlessly. We succumb to their designs. There is a universe of negligence and irresponsibility by the food industry, the pharmaceutical companies, unscrupulous physicians, dishonest merchants of hope and scammers. Their greed gets in our way and obstructs our better intentions.

As citizens and as the ones affected by the ills of society, we need to do two things: take care of ourselves and engage actively in demanding change from those who are threatening our existence . This is not a figurative assertion in a vacuum but a reality.

More than lifestyle modification, what is needed is a cultural change. If we become activists in defending our turf we will also comply with changes needed to assure good health. We all need to be in a mission to stay healthy, strong and fit, aging gracefully and coping with infirmities with a positive attitude. The mission in our life should not be rhetorical but rather an active engagement to pursue the purpose to be well and stay well. This entails two things: a transcendental elaboration of who we want to be emotionally and physically and vigorous action to support our ideas.

By connecting with the better part of ourselves, the quality of our lives will improve and we will fulfill the wish of marching through life with our self-esteem intact.

It is time for us to live a pastoral life, even if we live in a large, crowded city like New York or Chicago or Los Angeles.

It will be an invention of our imagination first; practical steps will help in configuring our own ideal habitat, full of positive connotations. We will create our own landscape in a crowded place; we will be romancing our commitment to be healthy. It will be our renaissance, the new woman, the new man.

Staying healthy is a strong commitment that can only be achieved with a more ample understanding of what it means. It is always entrenched with a physical and spiritual appreciation of the meaning of life, the purpose of living, understanding the obligation we have toward us and others and a strong dedication to share and give.

This is not a quixotic notion but it is true idealism that when executed will benefit you and humanity.

This devotion to serve others exists and is all around us. Others opposing our stand to live a healthy life in a sound environment are individuals and corporations with the purpose of enlarging their treasure chests. They should be recognized as our opponents; they are the forces we need to fight so we can prevail in the quest for health for us and our children. It is a civil conflict between one group that wants to impose their ways, regardless of the harm that may, in the long run, inflict and those of us who want to live a sensible life where the spiritual, social and physical values are above greed and materialistic aspirations.

They have the power that money gives, but we have the commitment that comes from our ideology; they are many, we are millions.

We are in the clinics filled with volunteers, in the schools where teachers are devoted to educate under any circumstances, in hospitals and laboratories where the scientists put all their efforts into meaningful research, in venues where artists advocate peace and prosperity, in organizations promoting us to be green and preserve the environment, in the decisions of those who give an organ to be transplanted to another, in the thousands of charities giving to the needy, in the countries where American surgeons go to provide services for free. Our force and our impetus is our commitment.

It all starts with helping yourself first so you can help others, like being in a plane when the oxygen mask comes down and you are supposed to adjust yours first so you can assist others.

In this idealized pastoral life, we will vow to:

Improve the environment

We all need to do our part. We can help in so many ways. Walk everywhere if distance allows it. Use a bicycle if safe. Climb up the stairs instead of taking the elevator. Recycle trash. Use our own bag when going to the market. Save water. Take short showers. The list goes on. Instructional material may be obtained free on the Internet and from public libraries and governmental and state agencies. Discuss with our friends and family what it means to go green, because sharing will make your endeavor meaningful. Pollution of our water, radioactivity, hazardous waste, soil contamination, excessive heat and noise are some of the contaminants that are affecting our health, producing neurological defects, degenerative disease and cancer, to name a few. So the first part of the mission is to prevent exposure to external agents that are toxic and lethal.

Improve eating habits

We have learned that food contains preservatives and chemicals that are toxic and the aggregate effect is the cause of many diseases. A recent epidemiological study showed that fish from rivers and reservoirs contain mercury, which is known to produce neurological damage and adversely affect pregnant women. The list is interminable. It is the cumulative effect that ends up being dangerous. The only way to overcome this problem is to consume food that is labeled organic and that we can find in the local farmers market or specialized food outlets. It is ironic that we call specialized those places that sell natural produce instead of the other way around. Supermarkets are now aware that there is a craving for all things that are natural and an aversion for what is artificial and have responded by creating special sections for organic food. If we all would patronize only markets that sell food without toxins or nasty chemicals, we could change the way the food industry operates.

Fruits and vegetables should be the base of our consumption, at least six servings a day. We can change the culture of cooking and become alchemists in the kitchen by making vegetables tasty and desirable. This will be our age of discovery. The veggie burger may become the staple of the nouveaux cuisine.

We should eat very little red meat and poultry. Fish (providing that we can be sure that is not contaminated) and vegetables will occupy center stage. A 6 oz. glass of red wine may complement our food. Bread and pasta should be occasional edibles. Whole grain, whole cereals are holy. Refined sugars are not fine.

We will not count calories but be conscious that when we finish our meal we should remain a little bit hungry. Salt, fat and sugar should be used at a minimum.

We should eat three full meals a day and a snack. The act of eating should be revered. Sitting at the table with our family or friends should be encouraged. Eating should be a momentous act, crucial as part of our daily routine. Being in a hurry, not having time to sit around the dining table denotes a failure in our lifestyle.

Fast food restaurants should not be supported, although they are part of our tradition. We probably have been going to them since we were kids. Fast food joints were many times a reward for our behavior. Visits to these places will be difficult to eradicate; after all, they offer succulent, tasty and cheap food, albeit unhealthy. They are the largest providers of noxious food and although some have incorporated some changes--for instance, by not cooking French fries in trans fats oil--they are now offering 24 oz. sodas containing more than 300 calories, not a commendable feature. What they are doing is disguising their many vices by practicing very few virtues.

Weight Control

We need to learn what our ideal weight is to carefully design a plan of action to achieve the goal of being on target. The Body Mass Index (BMI) is a better health indicator than weight. A BMI of 25 is normal and moving up or down up to 10 percent is acceptable, while more is harmful territory.

We discussed at length about the health implications of obesity. So now it is time to do something about it. Discard diet books; they are all unnecessary, unwanted and a waste of time and money. After a while they will be collecting dust on the shelves. Dietary guidelines are a different thing; they provide reliable data that conforms to the principles of science. Fad diets are to be ignored; books or articles that promise weight loss by ingenious manipulation of language and clever marketing have a short lifespan. There is no miracle diet; there are no Hollywood, Beverly Hills, Manhattan diets. Their promises and assurances to change your metabolism, your hormonal levels and your brain receptors are gimmicks. There is nothing better than a balanced, normal caloric diet with the right amount and quality of nutrients to improve our general health.

Appetite suppressants, although they may help initially, have undesirable side effects and cannot be taken for a long time without truly harming your body.

If it becomes hard for you to take the needed steps to achieve good health, there is plenty of help out there Nutritionists, help groups, physicians, psychologists, peer groups, addiction specialists, hospitals, churches, and counselors are always available to lend you a hand. Your medical insurance plan or your local hospital may have wellness program--just ask.

You can do it.

Enhanced Physical Activity

Walk, walk briskly if you can, jog, run, hike, bike, swim, dance-just do it.

Exercise should be part of a deliberate plan, performed ideally 7 days a week but no less than 5.

Exercise will keep you fit and healthy. The reward is immense. That is why we see hundreds of people in a gym performing all kinds of tasks to improve their health, their stamina, their flexibility. Most gyms have open windows that allow the passersby to appreciate the efforts of others. Now is our time.

It is our choice; it is our responsibility to strengthen our body. Doing what we have to do to stay healthy is part of a constellation of things that will help us to live better, to be happy. Working out our body is working out our mind.

Mens Sana in Corpore Sano, a healthy mind in a healthy body, could be paraphrased into a healthy body in a healthy mind, giving an indivisible connotation to the human being.

The time to educate ourselves about health is now. The time to do something about it is now.

Take as few medications as possible

As a physician, my premise has always been to prescribe as little medication as possible. Well, not always. Reglan (metoclopramide) was first introduced around 1964. This medication was effective in treating nausea and was also used to accelerate gastric emptying. It was a different class of medication and we gastroenterologists were excited to have such a drug in our therapeutic armamentarium. We used it extensively for many years with success and noticed that the drug had few side effects, none apparently very serious. I prescribed Reglan to one of my patients, along with other medications. When I saw the patient for follow-up four weeks later his GI symptoms had disappeared. He did not have any specific complaints but his girlfriend noticed that over the last 10 days he had become restless, had unusual behavior changes and his extremities were shaking. I was not sure about what was going on but asked him to stop all medications and come back in a week. I looked in the PDR book and learned that in very rare instances this medication may produce a syndrome called tardive dyskinesia. This made me reflect on the easiness we doctors have in filling prescriptions. It was a wake-up call and since then I have been very cautious and learned that less medications is better.

In our culture patients rely too much on medications and less in lifestyle modification. The problem is compounded by the eagerness of pharmaceutical companies to sell their products, and we end up having a society that loves to guzzle pills.

There are two types of situations that call for the consumption of medicinal products. One is an acute situation where medications are used to resolve a short-term problem. The other is when there are long-term situations that require prolonged intervention. **It is here when doctors and patients should exert extreme prudence. It is better to change our lifestyle than to be committed to take medications for the rest of our lives.**

We have previously discussed things we can do to limit medication intake while achieving the same level of comfort. Patients need to discuss with their doctors how to reduce their medication intake to a minimum.

About doctors and hospitals

Different physicians treat the same condition in different ways. This perplexing behavior is being addressed at different medical institutions by requiring the use of evidenced-based protocols that have been shown to save lives.

Patients put great faith in medicine, and this is understandable since they need an interlocutor when they are sick. Doctors ignore the premise that **patients get well in spite of them** and rush to administer treatment when what is called for is judicious observation and measured intervention. Many times physicians apply the latest approach, even when it has not been fully tested. That explains the mishaps with drugs and medical devices that are recalled by their manufacturers, but not before killing thousands of patients. Patients and families need to be aware of this and investigate what different hospitals are doing to improve quality of care and avoid mistakes. The Quality Department of each hospital can provide patients with this useful data.

About one million medical errors are committed every year in the US and 100,000 people die as a consequence. Hospitals are doing their best, in most cases, to track data and apply remedies to the situation by using root cause analysis methodology. You need to do your part. You should put the same effort into learning about doctors and hospitals that you exert when buying a car, in terms of efficiency, safety and performance. For this you need to be inquisitive and vocal. Speak up if you have any questions or doubts when you are in the hospital. Ask about medications you are getting, inquire about credentials of specialists that may have been assigned to your care, follow your intuition. Be pro-active. It is your health.

Use medical tools judiciously

When there are definitive, proven, time-tested treatments for a specific disease there is little dispute about treatment, which becomes conventional and accepted. Appendicitis calls for an appendectomy, a coronary artery blockage for angioplasty or bypass operation. Staph infection requires antibiotics and so on.

The problem is those conditions that are difficult to diagnose and treat. Here is when the worst of medicine starts playing a role. And the victim is always the patient.

The management of back pain is an example of the challenge that a chronic medical condition represents for patients and medical providers. The cause of back pain is difficult to ascertain, and treatment is usually ineffective, consuming and draining vast amounts of resources from the system. Solving the back pain dilemma and management of other chronic conditions will save enormous amounts of money and at the same time improve quality of care.

Jonah Lehrer tells in his book *How we decide* that treatment of back pain cost about 26 billion dollars a year, not counting workers' compensation and disability payments.

Back pain poses an economic burden because of lost work days, unnecessary diagnostic tests and the use of unproven, ineffectual treatments.

I can attest to this because I have suffered with back pain for many years. As a physician I believe that I judiciously used all known resources in an attempt to relieve my chronic back pain. I started by going to an orthopedic doctor. He ordered an MRI that showed minimal abnormalities. The radiologist interpreted that the findings were consistent with my age and could not clearly explain the cause for pain. Dr. Robert Wycoff, the radiologist, told me that most of the time radiologists have a hard time correlating findings and symptoms.

In fact, Lehrer mentions a study published in the *New England Journal of Medicine* that showed that images of the spinal region of ninety-eight people **without** back pain were reported as having 'serious problems' such as bulging, protruding or herniated discs in two-thirds of them. In 38 percent of these patients the MRI revealed multiple damaged discs and 90 percent exhibited some form of disc degeneration. My case, though, was the opposite. I had back pain and little findings. But the orthopedic doctor interpreted the scan as showing facet disease and ordered an MRI guided injection of corticosteroids into the facet joint. Wycoff told me that he could not assure me that it would relieve the pain, but I asked him to do it anyway. The pain relief lasted 36 hours, only to reappear later with the same intensity.

I was then referred to a rehabilitation center in Pasadena. The medical director, Dr. Sunil Hedge, put me in the hands of his best physical therapist. I underwent treatment for three months with some but not complete relief. About six months later my back pain started bothering me again. I read in the Health Section of the *Los Angeles Times* about an orthopedic doctor who opened a back pain center and treated patients successfully by non-surgical means. His sumptuous Beverly Hills Center was equipped with two kinds of machines that were aimed 'to open the intervertebral spaces.' I used the machine and in addition I received ultrasound treatment, heat and physical therapy. I abandoned treatment after four months because of lack of progress.

Other times I was treated for several months by acupuncturists and different chiropractors. I also resorted to Pilates and corporal massages. Nothing worked. Years later I went to see a different osteopath, who ordered 'dynamic' X-rays of the entire spine which consisted of images in different positions like flexion, extension and rotation of the cervical, dorsal and lumbar spine. They showed some subtle changes of the back (where I had pain) and severe right neural foraminal narrowing of the neck (where I have no pain). He prescribed anti-inflammatory and analgesic medication. I took them for 10 days, to no avail.

Years later I paid another visit to Wycoff to see if over the years my condition might have evolved. Reluctantly, we both decided that a new MRI with a new generation machine he had recently acquired was in order. The MRI was unchanged from the previous one but since I was on the table he proposed to attempt to control the pain with an epidural. I accepted. It did not work. My case is similar to millions of others who have pain originating either from the muscles, nerves, joints, or bones for which no definitive treatment exists. I decided that I was going to nurture my pain. I asked Sunil for advice about exercises that I could do and what things I should avoid. He recommended stretching and strengthening of core back muscles. I have been doing this for two years. My back pain is almost gone and I am able to function well.

My private insurance first and Medicare and my supplemental insurance later paid for all my diagnostic tests and treatments (with the exception of acupuncture and Pilates). I am a physician, supposedly a judicious and sensible man, who tried to get relief for my back pain; in the interim thousands of dollars were spent, first in diagnosing and then in management. Almost all the care for my back pain was ill-conceived. What was lacking was a sensible, experienced primary physician to guide me through the process. Now, in retrospect, I only needed one MRI, which would have shown the lack of significant pathology, and then sensible advice consisting of rest first followed by exercises and preventive measures to avoid aggravating the condition. Instead I saw multiple specialists and underwent many unnecessary tests and many unnecessary treatments; it was a costly, burdensome trip.

Lehrer explains the fact of poor utilization of resources in diagnosing and treating back pain as a failure in the rational method of decision-making. "Sometimes, more information and analysis can actually constrict thinking, making people understand less about what really is going on. Instead of focusing on the most pertinent variable--the percentage of patients who get better and experience less pain--doctors get sidetracked by the irrelevant MRI pictures. When it comes to treating back pain, this wrong-headed approach comes with serious costs," he wrote.

The prefrontal cortex is generally regarded as the rational center of the brain. "...it is a magnificent evolutionary development but must be used carefully. It can monitor thoughts and help evaluate emotions, but it can also paralyze, making a person forget the words of an aria or lose a trusty golf swing. When someone falls into the trap of spending much time about posters or about the details of an MRI image, the rational brain is being used in the wrong way. The prefrontal cortex can't handle so much complexity by itself," Lehrer explained.

My case, like those of millions with back pain, illustrates the poor utilization of resources that results in inordinate spending. And this concept can be extended to many other chronic conditions where effective treatments are elusive.

The rewards

Adopting a way of life, a consciousness of wellness, a means to take care of ourselves so we can give to others--in other words, shifting the paradigm of unawareness and lack of commitment to an inner pastoral life has a tremendous return on investment (as financiers like to call it). We need to become fully committed to a life of our invention; indifference toward what we do every day needs to be replaced with a sense of purpose in our life, a purpose that we should define, scrutinize and evaluate. Our daily routine needs to cease to be monotonous and dull; for this we need to change our habits in both the physical and spiritual spheres. We will replace our *laisse-faire* with a dedication to better ourselves. We will dedicate part of our time by actively disengaging from the vices of civilization, setting priorities, cultivating our relationships with friends and family, giving to others. It will be us who will dictate our behavior and not the corporations. Industrial food will be replaced by farm-grown edibles. Motion will substitute for stillness. We will use medicine intelligently. **Our wellbeing will be our recompense.**

APPENDIX 1:

Forty nutrients are required by the human body. Those that cannot be synthesized by the human body need to come from the outside and are called essential because their deficit causes significant illness and death, unless they are promptly replenished. The body requires proteins, small amounts of metabolizable carbohydrates, indigestible carbohydrate (fiber), nitrogen, minerals, vitamins and water to sustain life.

Proteins *are macromolecules composed of 20 different amino acids. They are arranged in variable order using information encoded in the genes. They are indispensable for growth, maintenance of body structure and function. They accomplish their task by arranging their small components in different sequences or by binding with other proteins. We can survive without fat but not without protein, so they must be included in every diet. They are a vital part of the cells and participate in every biological process. To give the reader an idea: insulin, which regulates blood sugar, is a protein; enzymes to digest food or act as the catalyst for any living cell process are proteins and without them we either get sick or die; immunity is protein dependent; muscle mass is a function of quantity and quality of certain proteins, to name only few of the functions. Proteins (complex molecules) are provided by food. Once they are ingested they are broken down in the gut into amino acids (simple molecules), absorbed and reconstituted, again as macromolecules, following different metabolic pathways. Men need about 56 grams of protein a day and women 45 to fulfill their body requirements, including energy. Some of these amino acids are converted into glucose, a concept that is important to keep in mind. Proteins are the mother of all bodily functions and like almost all mothers, we should hold them in high regard. Each gram of protein renders four calories.*

The story is different for fat. ***Fat*** *provides 9 calories per gram, is the more concentrated source of food energy and, like dietary carbohydrates, can support protein synthesis (remember that amino acids can be converted into glucose,* which means that protein, fat and carbohydrates can balance for each other). This is another mechanism by which the body can compensate for its deficits; it will be as if a car could use ethanol or diesel when regular gasoline is not available.

We can live with little fat; the only essential fatty acid we need is linoleic acid, providing that our energetic needs are fulfilled by other nutrients. (A word of caution--what science claims as good today may be bad tomorrow. In August 2009 an article published in the British medical journal GUT showed that **excessive** dietary linoleic acid increases the incidence of ulcerative colitis). Yet it is unwise to eliminate fat completely from the diet because it plays an important role in maintaining body temperature, promoting healthy cell function and preserving healthy skin and hair. Fats are supplied by animals or plants. The American diet contains 40 percent of calories as fat; the recommended dose is 30 percent, and even less is safe and well tolerated. Fat comes from different sources and is present in practically every foodstuff we eat, some of which are obvious, like butter and oil, and others not apparent, like fish or yogurt.

Fat is composed of cholesterol and fatty acids, which can be saturated, monounsaturated and polyunsaturated. Saturated fats are bad because they increase cholesterol, while the other two have the opposite effect. Eating too much fat leads to infirmity and in the long run is lethal. A deficiency of linoleic acid impairs wound healing and produces dermatitis and weight loss.

Cholesterol occupies a special place in our culture and today the word has a negative connotation. It is a topic of conversation when discussing health matters. It has a symbolic meaning, appearing to be the source of all ills, a thief stealing our wellbeing, an outlaw maiming us little by little. But wait, cholesterol is also a good guy, keeping us alive, making sure that vitamins are absorbed and cells have the capacity to do their work, maintaining conduction in nerve cells intact and responsible for manufacturing bile acids and hormones among other multiple functions.

Cholesterol at the right concentration is our savior, at the wrong one our enemy.

Cholesterol comes from two sources. One, called endogenous, comes from the machinations of our body (metabolism). The other, called exogenous, is the one contained in food. If we eat too much cholesterol our body will partially shut off the production of the endogenous counterpart. The recommended amount of dietary cholesterol is 300 mg or less per day to avoid excessive serum concentration, which is associated with atherosclerosis.

Cholesterol is present in animal fat but not in vegetables. Flax seeds and peanuts contain phytosterols, which appear to lower serum cholesterol. Cholesterol is transported by lipoproteins, which they carry to certain tissues. For our purposes, it is important to recognize two types of lipoproteins, low density (LDL) and high density (HDL). LDL is the bad lipoprotein; we call it bad because it transports large amounts of cholesterol. It is like a carrier delivering stuff to wrong places. The LDL, after some metabolic transformation, is responsible for the formation of atherosclerotic plaque, which leads to stroke, myocardial infarction and peripheral vascular disease, among many other serious medical problems. The High Density Lipoprotein (HDL) is the good cholesterol. When it comes to HDL, more is better and less is worse. HDL is considered the good one because it transports cholesterol to the liver, where it can be eliminated from the body. Independent of the concentration of LDL, low HDL can by itself lead to hardening of the arteries. It is as important to measure total cholesterol level in the blood as it is to know the concentration of LDL and HDL. In other words, don't be fooled by a "normal" cholesterol figure when the ratio between the good and bad components is reversed. Cholesterol was not of medical interest in the early 1940s; in fact, physicians somewhat ignored it until 1985, when it became a medical concern. Multiple studies have shown the link with different medical conditions, although in the right concentration it is an essential component of the human body, present in cell membranes and bile, precursor of liposoluble vitamins and steroid hormones, to name only a few of its vital functions.

Carbohydrates, also known as sugars, are the other source of energy. They are not an indispensable part of the diet because the human body can obtain its entire energy requirement from protein and fat. But when we fast, the lack of carbohydrates leads to ketosis, a severe metabolic disorder. In practice most dietary energy is provided by carbohydrates. Carbohydrates contain 3.75 calories per gram. The recommended dietary allowance is 55 to 60 percent of total calories in the diet. There are three types of sugars. The basic carbohydrate is a monosaccharide- one unit- (like glucose, galactose, xylose, ribose and fructose); disaccharide - two units- (like lactose present in milk; sucrose or table sugar and maltose present in vegetables and beer) and complex carbohydrates –multiple units- (like starches present in legumes, vegetables, whole-grain bread and cereals and fiber, which is an indigestible carbohydrate).

Monosaccharides (MS) can be connected together and form oligosaccharides (OS) or polysacchararides (PS). When they are not needed they are stored in the liver and muscle cells in the form of glycogen and released upon demand. To be more graphic, they are like a chain where one link is a MS, two or three are OS and more are PS. The more links, the better in terms of their ability to provide strength.

Complex molecules, in order to be absorbed, need to be converted to simple molecules (monosaccharides). This is done by enzymes present in the small bowel; for instance, lactose is converted into glucose and galactose by lactase before being able to enter the bloodstream. When there is a lactase deficiency, the larger lactose molecule cannot be absorbed and its mere presence pulls water from the body into the lumen of the intestine and produces diarrhea. Sugars are simple carbohydrates. Simple and refined sugars provide calories but no vitamins, minerals or fiber and because of this they are called "empty calories." They promote obesity. They are present in candies, table sugar and sugary drinks, among others.

In Essence: Most of the foods we consume come in large particles, which are converted into small ones by the action of digestive enzymes. After their breakdown into small units, they are absorbed in the small intestine and later reconstituted into larger ones, at which time they are stored in different parts of the body and released upon demand. In addition, proteins may become sugars, and sugars and fat may compensate for each other.

Other essential nutrients obtained from the diet are **vitamins** and **minerals**. They are not synthesized by the human body. Their deficiency may cause irreparable body damage and death. They have diverse biochemical functions like in the formation of hormones (vitamin D), antioxidants (vitamin E) and regulators of cell and tissue growth, among many others. Minerals are the chemical elements essential in supporting biochemical reactions to maintain optimal health and are easily obtained with a basic diet, but when there is an ailment that impairs its absorption or excretion, the end result can rapidly produce the demise of a person, for instance in the case of intractable diarrhea where the loss of a mineral like potassium (which is essential in maintaining proper heart function) can produce a fatal arrhythmia unless the problem is promptly corrected.

The bottom line is that we get all we need to survive through what we eat, but what we eat comes in different forms and qualities. Sugars and fats are not the same, although they both provide needed energy. To be more explicit: just like the performance of an engine varies if it runs on gas with different octanes, electricity, alcohol or diesel, our body will function as well or as badly, depending on what we use as nourishment.

APPENDIX 2: FOOD GROUPS

A brief classification of what we eat is useful as a memory aid and once it becomes embedded in us, we may automatically think about food in a different way; for example, whole grains are excellent nutrients while refined are not that good. Vegetables of all colors, flavors, shapes and aromas are good, very good. Meats are both precious and unworthy because although they provide nourishment, they are also the source of bad cholesterol.

Grains: there are two types, whole and refined. Whole grain contains the whole kernel and contains iron, vitamin B and fiber, while refined does not unless enriched with added vitamin and iron.

Examples of whole grains are: brown rice, oatmeal, cracked wheat, whole cereal flakes, whole wheat pasta, wild rice, buckwheat, whole wheat tortillas, and whole wheat bread, among others. Some of the grain products contain bran, which provides fiber.

Refined grains, unless labeled otherwise, include cornbread, white bread, spaghetti, macaroni, flour or corn tortillas, crackers, noodles and white rice. The daily recommendations are from 3 to 8 oz., depending on age and sex. Those who exercise may eat more. Always go for the wholesome whole grain and avoid the refined one.

Vegetables: Veggies come in many forms: raw, juices, cooked, canned, fresh, and frozen. It is always better to eat them fresh because the others, in the process of preserving them or making them more palatable, may contain undesirable chemicals. There are several subgroups of vegetables.

Dark Green: Broccoli, mesclun, romaine lettuce, spinach, watercress, turnip green, dark green leafy lettuce, collard green, mustard green and bok choy; all full of valuable nutrients, vitamins and antioxidants.

Orange vegetables: acorn squash, butternut squash, carrots, hubbard squash, pumpkin and sweet potatoes.

Starchy vegetables: corn, green peas, green lima beans and potatoes.

Others: artichokes, asparagus, bean sprouts, beets, Brussels sprouts, cabbage, cauliflower, celery, cucumbers, eggplants, green beans, green or red peppers, iceberg lettuce, mushrooms, okra, onions, parsnips, tomatoes, turnips, wax beans and zucchini. The desirable amount is 1 to 3 cups a day, always depending on age, sex and level of physical activity. They are usually low in calories and nutritionally sound.

Fruits: *There are different groups, from berries to nectarines to melons and in between. They all have enormous health benefits and when they are part of a healthy diet, they reduce the risk of some chronic diseases. They are naturally low in fat, sodium and calories and none have cholesterol. They contain minerals and vitamins.*

Milk, yogurt and cheese: *They are good sources of calcium.*

Milk group choices should be fat free or low fat. Cheese comes in all forms, shapes, and flavors and is an excellent source of protein, phosphorus, and calcium, but it also contains variable amounts of saturated fat and salt, for which reason it should be restricted to certain limits. Yogurt is rich in protein and B vitamins, has better nutritional value than milk and can be consumed by people who have moderate lactose intolerance. In addition, it has Lactobacillus acidophilus that appears to prevent Candida vulvovaginitis and antibiotic-associated diarrhea.

Meats: *Includes beef, game, poultry and fish and all of its internal organs like liver, brain, pancreas and the like. Meats are excellent sources of proteins, vitamins and minerals but they also contain high saturated fat and cholesterol, which makes them less desirable, so in order to be beneficial they have to be lean and should be consumed sparingly. Fish are permissible, especially herring, trout and salmon, which in addition to good proteins contain omega-3 fatty acids, which appear to reduce the risk of cardiovascular disease.*

Industrialization of meats in general has made them unreliable, with the exception of some that are carefully treated during the process of production. Producers can manipulate the whole spectrum of animals using hormones to accelerate muscle growth, sedatives to increase weight, antibiotics to improve growth rate, and genetic manipulation to increase commercial value by shortening breeding program so they end up tasting good but hiding noxious elements. Another problem with meat is that not infrequently it is contaminated with bacteria coming from either the animals or during the growing phase, processing, storing, harvesting or shipping of the animals, as well during the final preparation of a meal. In fact, about 76 million people may contract a foodborne illness every year and 5000 may die. The common contaminants are Salmonella, Shigella, E. coli 017-H7, viruses and parasites.

Eggs: Egg yolk contains cholesterol and egg whites do not. They are an excellent source of proteins. The taste of the eggs depends on the diet of the birds and conditions during storage. They are at times contaminated, especially with salmonella, and because of this it is important to cook them thoroughly and discard them if not eaten 2 weeks after refrigeration. Infections arise from a weakened shell and can also be prevented by vaccinating poultry. Because the yolk contains saturated fat, there is a controversy whether eggs may affect adversely the health of individuals, mainly those with high cholesterol and diabetes. Some nutritionists claim that one or two eggs a day may be consumed safely, while others advocate no eggs at all. Common sense, validated by some science, suggests that eating two eggs a week may be beneficial, since they are an excellent source of proteins, calcium, vitamins, phosphorus, potassium, iron and choline (important during pregnancy and nursing), as well as folic acid.

Dry beans and peas: They contain vitamins A, C, E, B, iron and magnesium. There is a large variety of beans, including green, black, white, yellow, soybean, fava, lime and pinto, to name some of the 37 listed beans.

Nut and seeds: These are good sources of essential fatty acids and vitamin E. Flax, walnuts, sunflower seeds, almonds and hazelnuts are the preferred ones. They are a good substitute for unhealthy snacks, since they are also a source of Omega 3-fatty acids and helpful in reducing LDL (the bad lipoprotein).

Oils: Oils come from animals or plants. Vegetable oils are liquid at room temperature and used for cooking or as food dressings. They come from different plants and most have no cholesterol and are high on the desirable monounsaturated and polyunsaturated fats. Animal oils are solid at room temperature and, like pork fat (lard) and beef fat (tallow, suet), should be discarded from the American diet. They are still being used in most of the junk food eateries because they are cheap and tasty.

Coconut oil and palm kernel oil are high in saturated fat and should be considered in the category of solid fat.

In Summary: As simple or as complicated as it sounds, knowing the above facts outlined in the preceding seven pages may empower you to eat right and will help to keep your body healthy, combat infirmities and give you the wellbeing that we all aspire to. That is the first step. Next, you will learn to avoid external forces that are conniving, purposely or not, to maim you physically and emotionally.